Anesthesia

Editors

DAVID W. TODD
ROBERT C. BOSACK

ORAL AND MAXILLOFACIAL SURGERY CLINICS OF NORTH AMERICA

www.oralmaxsurgery.theclinics.com

Consulting Editor
RICHARD H. HAUG

May 2018 • Volume 30 • Number 2

ELSEVIER

1600 John F. Kennedy Boulevard • Suite 1800 • Philadelphia, Pennsylvania, 19103-2899

http://www.oralmaxsurgery.theclinics.com

**ORAL AND MAXILLOFACIAL SURGERY CLINICS OF NORTH AMERICA Volume 30, Number 2
May 2018 ISSN 1042-3699, ISBN-13: 978-0-323-58370-1**

Editor: John Vassallo; j.vassallo@elsevier.com
Developmental Editor: Laura Fisher

Oral and Maxillofacial Surgery Clinics of North America (ISSN 1042-3699) is published quarterly by Elsevier Inc., 360 Park Avenue South, New York, NY 10010-1710. Months of issue are February, May, August, and November. Business and Editorial Offices: 1600 John F. Kennedy Blvd., Suite 1800, Philadelphia, PA 19103-2899. Periodicals postage paid at New York, NY and additional mailing offices. Subscription prices are $393.00 per year for US individuals, $686.00 per year for US institutions, $100.00 per year for US students and residents, $464.00 per year for Canadian individuals, $822.00 per year for Canadian institutions, $520.00 per year for international individuals, $822.00 per year for international institutions and $235.00 per year for Canadian and foreign students/residents. To receive student/resident rate, orders must be accompanied by name or affiliated institution, date of term, and the *signature* of program/residency coordinator on institution letterhead. Orders will be billed at individual rate until proof of status is received. Foreign air speed delivery is included in all *Clinics* subscription prices. All prices are subject to change without notice. **POSTMASTER:** Send address changes to *Oral and Maxillofacial Surgery Clinics of North America,* Elsevier Periodicals **Customer Service, 11830 Westline Industrial Drive, St. Louis, MO 63146. Tel: 1-800-654-2452 (U.S. and Canada); 314-447-8871 (outside U.S. and Canada). Fax: 314-447-8029. E-mail: journals customerservice-usa@elsevier.com (for print support); journalsonlinesupport-usa@elsevier.com (for online support).**

Reprints. For copies of 100 or more, of articles in this publication, please contact the Commercial Reprints Department, Elsevier Inc., 360 Park Avenue South, New York, NY 10010-1710. Tel.: 212-633-3874; Fax: 212-633-3820; Email: reprints@elsevier.com.

Oral and Maxillofacial Surgery Clinics of North America is covered in *MEDLINE/PubMed (Index Medicus), Science Citation Index Expanded (SciSearch®), Journal Citation Reports/Science Edition,* and *Current Contents®/Clinical Medicine.*

Contributors

CONSULTING EDITOR

RICHARD H. HAUG, DDS[†]
Professor and Chief, Oral Maxillofacial Surgery, Carolinas Medical Center, Charlotte, North Carolina, USA

EDITORS

DAVID W. TODD, DMD, MD
Private Practice, Lakewood, New York

ROBERT C. BOSACK, DDS
Private Practice, Orland Park, Illinois; Clinical Assistant Professor, University of Illinois at Chicago, College of Dentistry, Chicago, Illinois

AUTHORS

ROBERT C. BOSACK, DDS
Private Practice, Orland Park, Illinois; Clinical Assistant Professor, University of Illinois at Chicago, College of Dentistry, Chicago, Illinois

JASON W. BRADY, DMD
Attending, Department of Dental Anesthesia, NYU Langone Hospital, Brooklyn, New York; Orthodontics and General Practice Residency, Adjunct Faculty, Division of Endodontics, Herman Ostrow School of Dentistry of USC, Los Angeles, California

STEPHANIE J. DREW, DMD, FACS
Associate Clinical Professor, Division of Oral and Maxillofacial Surgery, Emory University School of Medicine, Atlanta, Georgia

KYLE J. KRAMER, DDS, MS
Clinical Assistant Professor, Department of Oral Surgery and Hospital Dentistry, Indiana University School of Dentistry, Indianapolis, Indiana

DEEPAK G. KRISHNAN, DDS, FACS
Associate Professor of Surgery and Residency Program Director, Division of Oral Maxillofacial Surgery, Department of Surgery, University of Cincinnati, Cincinnati, Ohio

STUART LIEBLICH, DMD
Clinical Professor, University of Connecticut School of Dental Medicine, Farmington, Connecticut; Private Practice, Avon Oral and Maxillofacial Surgery, Avon, Connecticut

CHIRAG M. PATEL, DMD, MD
Assistant Clinical Professor, Department of Oral and Maxillofacial Surgery, University of California, San Francisco School of Dentistry, San Francisco, California

MICHAEL R. RAGAN, DMD, JD, LLM
Adjunct Professor, Department of Oral and Maxillofacial Surgery, Nova Southeastern University, College of Dental Medicine, Fort Lauderdale, Florida

CLIVE RAYNER, DMD
Private Practice, Orange Park, Florida

RICHARD C. ROBERT, DDS, MS
Clinical Professor, Department of Oral and Maxillofacial Surgery, University of California, San Francisco School of Dentistry, San Francisco, California

[†]Deceased

JOHN J. SCHAEFER III, MD
Lewis W. Haskell Blackman Endowed Chair,
Professor, Department of Anesthesia
and Perioperative Medicine, Medical
University of South Carolina, Charleston,
South Carolina

ALLAN SCHWARTZ, DDS, CRNA
Assistant Professor, Department of Periodontics,
Center for Advanced Dental Education, Saint
Louis University, St Louis, Missouri

DAVID W. TODD, DMD, MD
Private Practice, Lakewood, New York

Contents

> Efficient responses to emergencies in the oral and maxillofacial surgery office require preparation, communication, and thorough documentation of the event and response. The concept of team anesthesia is showcased with these efforts. Emergency medical services training and response times vary greatly. The oral and maxillofacial surgery office should be prepared to manage the patient for at least 15 minutes after making the call to 911. Patient outcomes are optimized when providers work together to manage and transport the patient. Oral and maxillofacial surgery offices should develop and rehearse emergency plans and coordinate these protocols with local emergency medical services teams.

> Provision of an outpatient anesthetic requires careful review of the patient's medical history along with salient aspects of the physical examination. The oral and maxillofacial surgeon may need to consult with the patient's medical providers to gain an understanding of the patient's potential risks for an adverse event. This article reviews key aspects of the patient evaluation so that an informed determination of suitability for an office anesthetic can be made.

> The model for oral and maxillofacial surgery (OMFS) delivery of office-based, open airway anesthesia has morphed from the operator-anesthetist to the delivery of team anesthesia, supporting a widespread focus on organizational aspects of the delivery of care. The training, continuing education, and coordination of a diverse anesthesia team provide a system to improve the safety and efficacy of anesthesia delivery. The hallmarks of this system include communication, checks and balances, monitoring, team dynamics, protocols, emergency scenario preparation and rehearsal, and crisis resource management during an emergent situation. This system contributes to and continually supports a culture of safety in the OMFS office.

> Oral and maxillofacial surgeons have a variety of anesthetic agents that can be used to provide anesthesia safely and efficiently in the office-based environment.

However, it is critical to have a thorough understanding of the particulars for each agent. Commonly used anesthetic agents, administered either individually or in combination, include diazepam, midazolam, propofol, ketamine, opioid agonists such as fentanyl or remifentanil, dexmedetomidine, and inhalational agents, including nitrous oxide and sevoflurane. These agents help provide extreme flexibility for those creating an individualized anesthetic plan that also balances the patient's history and the anticipated surgical plan to maximize success.

Owing to wide variation in patient responses, both intended and adverse, it is impossible to successfully sedate all patients. Choosing the right drug and dose regimen can be challenging, especially in patients who are naive to anesthesia. Underdosing can lead to pain perception, patient movement and combativeness, awareness with recall, and the sympathetic neuroendocrine stress response. Overdosing can lead to unintended loss of upper airway tone, hypoventilation/apnea, adverse cardiovascular changes, and prolonged sedation (with its attendant problems).

Pediatric patients present to the oral and maxillofacial surgeon for surgical services that can be performed safely and efficiently. Children and parents tend to be anxious; achieving cooperation is paramount for successful procedures. Several techniques can be used to alleviate anxiety and provide analgesia and anesthesia. This article outlines the anatomy and physiology of children and the preoperative anesthetic preparation and techniques unique to pediatric anesthesia. It discusses standards in training in pediatric anesthesia and current recommendations for monitoring. Management of children with autism spectrum disorders and attention deficit hyperactivity disorders highlights special considerations in the management of these children.

An effective office emergency preparedness plan for the oral and maxillofacial surgery office can be developed through the use of well-designed checklists, cognitive aids, and regularly scheduled in situ simulations with debriefings. To achieve this goal, the hierarchal culture of medicine and dentistry must be overcome and an inclusive team concept embraced by all members of the staff. Technologic advancements in office automation now make it possible to create interactive cognitive aids. These enhance office emergency training and provide a means for more rapid retrieval of essential information and guidance during both simulations and a real crisis.

Patient safety in dental anesthesia has been called into question in recent years. Simulation training has been proposed and developed as one possibility for increasing preparedness and training in cases of adverse events in dental anesthesia. This article presents an overview of the challenges of patient safety in dental anesthesia and how to address them with simulation training. The American Association of Oral and Maxillofacial Surgeons simulation program is unique in its potential to become a standardized, validated competency course with objective grading criteria, mastery-based cooperative learning model, and low facilitator to participant ratio, leading to a practical delivery cost structure.

Airway Management for the Oral Surgery Patient   207

Allan Schwartz

This article discusses anesthesia assessment concepts related to airway evaluation and airway maintenance for safe and reliable selection of either open system (entrainment of room air) or closed system (no entrainment of room air) airway devices, which can be used during office-based oral surgical procedures, depending on the needs of a patient. Dental facial and oral structures are integral to an anesthetist's preoperative patient evaluation before surgery. The preoperative medical history and physical examination as well as the nature of the oral surgical procedure affect the selection of a proper and safe airway device.

Anesthetic Pump Techniques Versus the Intermittent Bolus: What the Oral Surgeon Needs to Know   227

Richard C. Robert and Chirag M. Patel

The most popular agents in use for office-based anesthesia are propofol, ketamine, and remifentanil, which have the desirable properties of rapid onset and short duration of action. A useful parameter in assessing these agents is the context-sensitive half-time. These anesthetic agents demonstrate relatively low, flat plots compared with older agents. For delivery of intravenous anesthetics, oral and maxillofacial surgeons have relied on small incremental boluses with great success. However, relatively simple syringe infusion pumps can provide an even "smoother" anesthetic. This article familiarizes oral and maxillofacial surgeons with the advantages of infusion pumps and provides examples of their use.

ORAL AND MAXILLOFACIAL SURGERY CLINICS OF NORTH AMERICA

THE CLINICS ARE NOW AVAILABLE ONLINE!
Access your subscription at:
www.theclinics.com

n Memoriam

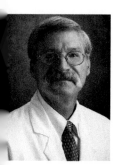

Richard H. Haug, DDS
Consulting Editor

Richard H. Haug, DDS, the Consulting Editor of the *Oral and Maxillofacial Surgery Clinics of North America* and *Atlas of the Oral and Maxillofacial Surgery Clinics of North America*, passed away Thursday, January 25, 2018 after a short illness. He was surrounded by his family and friends.

Dr Haug was an Oral and Maxillofacial Surgeon at Carolinas Center for Oral Health within the Department of Oral Medicine in Charlotte, North Carolina for the past nine years. He provided specialized care for a wide range of medically complex patients. His commitment and compassion to patient care, teaching, and research were nothing short of exemplary and are the standard for all to strive. He was beloved by his patients, the faculty, residents, and staff within Oral Medicine, Oral Surgery, and many others throughout the Carolinas HealthCare System.

Rich graduated with honors from SUNY Stony Brook in 1980 and had academic appointments in Stony Brook, New York, Cleveland, Ohio, and Lexington, Kentucky before joining Carolinas Center for Oral Health in 2009. His career was distinguished by many honors, including The Daniel M. Laskin Award (for the best paper in the *Journal of Oral and Maxillofacial Surgery of North America* in 2002) and The Donald B. Osbon Outstanding Educator Award, presented at the AAOMS 89th Annual Meeting in Honolulu, Hawaii.

Rich was editor of *Oral and Maxillofacial Surgery Clinics of North America* for over 15 years and was personally involved in and integral to the success of every issue he edited (more than 60): from initial conception of the topic, to inviting the guest editor(s), to reviewing thousands of page proofs. His demand for quality and expertise in every topic and guest editor has built and sustained the excellent reputation of the series all these years.

Rich was a Mason his entire adult life and was active in local lodges in every city he resided in for years. In lieu of flowers, he had requested that his friends and colleagues consider donating to the Masonic Home for Children in Oxford, North Carolina (http://mhc-oxford.org/) in his memory.

He will be greatly missed by us all.

Michael T. Brennan, DDS, MHS
Department of Oral Medicine
Carolinas Medical Center
Charlotte, NC 28203, USA

John Vassallo
Editor, Oral and Maxillofacial Surgery Clinics of North America

E-mail address:
Mike.Brennan@carolinashealthcare.org

Preface

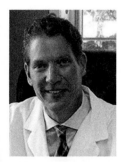 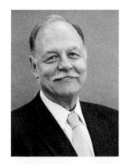

David W. Todd, DMD, MD   Robert C. Bosack, DDS
Editors

We are pleased to welcome you to this timely issue of *Oral and Maxillofacial Surgery Clinics of North America* devoted exclusively to office-based anesthesia. This topic reinforces and complements the May 2017 issue on Patient Safety.

Office-based anesthesia is a core component of the oral and maxillofacial surgery (OMFS) practice, and this privilege readily differentiates the OMFS specialty from all other dental and medical specialties. The specialized training goes well beyond a 5-6 month operating room anesthesia rotation, as OMFS residents complete a variety of complementary rotations in surgery, medicine, intensive care, and office-based clinical anesthesia. This training, together with full pallet of continuing education programs, dedicated exclusively to anesthesia, enhances the ability of the OMFS to appropriately select patients and open airway anesthetic techniques, permitting the anxiety and pain-free completion of a wide range of surgical procedures. Also unique to the OMFS practice is the adaption of what we refer to as *team anesthesia*, where formally trained anesthesia assistants help to monitor the patient and provide basic airway maneuvers. Despite an enviable safety record, there are critics of our anesthesia model and every oral and maxillofacial surgeon (OMS) must ensure that their practice has in place a culture of safety and that their anesthesia team is well trained in the unique aspects of anesthesia delivery in the office environment.

This issue of *Oral and Maxillofacial Surgery Clinics of North America* is dedicated to updating the OMS on many aspects of office-based anesthesia practice. This issue includes reviews of assistant training, techniques and agents, patient safety concepts, and what to do when things go wrong. In addition, this issue includes for the first time a description of the American Association of Oral and Maxillofacial Surgeons simulation program.

We would like to extend our gratitude to Mr John Vassallo and his staff at Elsevier for their help in constructing this valuable resource.

David W. Todd, DMD, MD
Private Practice
120 Southwestern Drive
Lakewood, NY 14750, USA

Robert C. Bosack, DDS
Private Practice
16011 S. 108th Avenue
Orland Park, IL 60467, USA

University of Illinois at Chicago
College of Dentistry
Chicago, IL 60612, USA

E-mail addresses:
David@dwtodd.com (D.W. Todd)
r.bosack@comcast.net (R.C. Bosack)

Oral Maxillofacial Surg Clin N Am 30 (2018) xi
https://doi.org/10.1016/j.coms.2018.02.003
1042-3699/18/© 2018 Published by Elsevier Inc.

Are You Ready for Emergency Medical Services in Your Oral and Maxillofacial Surgery Office?

Clive Rayner, DMD[a],*, Michael R. Ragan, DMD, JD, LLM[b,1]

KEYWORDS

- EMS • Medicolegal • Emergency preparedness • Office-based anesthesia
- Crisis resource management

KEY POINTS

- Oral and maxillofacial surgery practices should be familiar with the functionality of their local emergency medical services system (response time, training/ability of responders, onsite hierarchy, and logistics of patient transport).
- Emergency medical services skills and response times can vary; the oral and maxillofacial surgery office should be prepared to stabilize the patient for at least 15 minutes.
- The office should be prepared to manage the patient until Emergency medical services arrives and to coordinate care among the various teams.
- Emergency medical services teams usually follow specific standing medical orders from their medical directors that can conflict with the wishes of the oral and maxillofacial surgeon.
- The oral and maxillofacial surgery office should be prepared to reassert management of the emergency should emergency medical services fail to successfully manage the situation.

INTRODUCTION

Emergency medical services (EMS) provide out-of-hospital acute medical care and transport to definitive care, among other services. Although the frequency of true medical or anesthetic emergencies are currently not tracked, it is likely, and perhaps inevitable, that all oral and maxillofacial surgery (OMS) offices will experience at least 1 emergent situation requiring EMS assistance or transport during their practice lifetime. Because the training, experience, and ability to identify and manage these emergencies are quite variable, the ongoing challenge of anticipation, preparation, and management of emergencies must be continually addressed. This article focuses on the mechanics, interplay, and outcomes once "activate EMS" is reached in any given algorithm.

THE CALL TO 911

The call to 911 provides access to police, fire, ambulance services and EMS via a Public Safety Answering Point (PSAP).[1,2]

The call to 911 is not a sign of weakness, inability, embarrassment, or failure. Rather, it reinforces the OMS's commitment to all patients

Disclosure Statement: The opinions expressed herein are those of the authors, and do not represent legal or medical/dental advice. Neither author has any conflict of interest to disclose.

[a] Private Practice, 2301 Park Avenue #101, Orange Park, FL 32073, USA; [b] Department of Oral and Maxillofacial Surgery, Nova Southeastern University, College of Dental Medicine, 3301 College Avenue, Fort Lauderdale, FL 33314, USA
[1] 19 West Flagler Street Suite 211, Miami, FL 33131.
* Corresponding author.
E-mail address: jawdoc00@gmail.com

to provide the best possible care, regardless of circumstance. It is both recognized and accepted that patient responses can be unpredictable, and there are established limits to both diagnostic and treatment modalities that are available in any OMS facility. Contacting EMS remains a judgment call on the part of the OMS. However, regardless of circumstance, if events occur that will prevent the patient from returning home for independent living, the call for (at minimum) transport to another facility should not be delayed.

Throughout the United States, there are many different methods of administration, operation, and dispatch of these services, which also vary based on geographic and political boundaries. An example would be a jurisdiction that operates its own PSAP, but not EMS. As a result, there can be overlapping jurisdictions, which often result in delays of longer than 1 minute as information is routed or transferred from 1 jurisdiction to another, or 1 jurisdiction to an independent EMS. In such cases, it is entirely possible to have a 911 call routed to a general information number, resulting in even further delays. Similar delays can occur when the local EMS is occupied with other events; in this instance, a neighboring jurisdiction will be subsequently contacted. An understanding of the structure of these services in any locale, thus, becomes most important in cases of airway compromise, where minutes can make the difference between life and death.

Approximately 80% of 911 calls now come from cell phones, which prevent autolocation of the call, a convenient and time-saving safety feature that is enabled when calls are made from a traditional land line. Autolocation will identify a time of call, name, number, and address of the caller, which typically is voice verified to ensure the accuracy of this information. Additionally, all calls to 911 are recorded. The medicolegal consequences of this recording are obvious, because these phone calls are considered to be a legal document. It behooves each office to learn and understand the specifics of making this call, such that the caller remain calm, organized, and complete in the conveyance of information.

In the proposed "Next-Generation 911" environment, the public will be able to make voice, text, or video emergency calls from any communication device via Internet protocol-based networks. The new infrastructure will also support national networking of 911 services, and transfer of emergency calls to other PSAPs, including any accompanying data.[3]

Surprisingly, the educational requirements for an emergency dispatcher are minimal and optional: for example, a 24-hour course in which students are trained to gather information about the nature of the emergency and patient location followed by triage and dispatch to the appropriate EMS resource.

OMS offices should ideally develop formal written protocols that describe the specifics of contacting EMS. Specific roles should be preassigned, and instructions given as to who will make the call, and what will be said and revealed to the dispatcher, who typically is trained to follow caller interrogation protocol. This protocol should be reviewed and rehearsed regularly, as part of a larger, comprehensive, written office emergency protocol that also includes procedures and staff roles in responding to an office medical emergency.[4–7] The following questions can be anticipated during this recorded call:

1. 911, What are you reporting?
2. What is the address of the patient?
3. What is the patient's age and gender
4. What telephone number are you calling from?
5. What is your name?
6. Is the patient conscious (awake, conversant, and coherent)?
7. Is the person breathing normally?

If a formal interrogation protocol is not followed, the OMS team should tell the EMS dispatcher the nature of the emergency and, if it is life threatening, they should immediately say so (eg, "the patient is unconscious and not breathing" or "the patient is having a bronchospasm") and specifically request advanced life support (ALS) EMS immediately. Again, the name and address of the office and nearby landmarks to assist in locating the office should be tendered, as well as the nature of ongoing therapy and the telephone number of the office.

The dispatcher will usually ask the caller to stay on the phone, which may occupy the attention of an office staff member whose assistance can often be better used in the ongoing emergency therapy. Occasionally, the dispatcher may have formal written guidelines to verbally "coach" the caller through emergency cardiopulmonary resuscitation or obstructed airway sequences, but there are no guidelines for the dispatcher to offer to the OMS team relating to the management of an anesthetic emergency. As such, little may be gained by staying on the line with the dispatcher, other than to track the arrival of EMS. It is prudent to ask the dispatcher, "How long until advanced life support (paramedics) can be here?" Roam phones can prove to be invaluable in these instances.

The time that the call is made must be documented.

EMERGENCY MEDICAL SERVICES RESPONSE TIMES

EMS response times vary widely, from approximately 5 minutes in Seattle to approximately 12 minutes in New York City.[8,9] Although there are no national standards or requirements, the US national stated goal (by the National Fire Prevention Association) for EMS response to life-threatening emergencies is less than 9 minutes 90% of the time, and that is defined as the time needed "to deploy at the first responder level with AED [automated external defibrillator] or higher treatment level,"[10,11] however, this objective is rarely achieved. As call volumes increase and resources and funding fail to keep pace, even large EMS systems struggle to meet these standards. Sources differ, but the US average is reported to be approximately 10.5 minutes, with considerable variance and a possibility that up to 10% of the calls may take more than 20 minutes. Rural and congested urban areas have the longest response times.[12–15] It is important to note that this "time" from call to first responder presence at the patient's side is not measured in any standardized fashion, with each call center using their own methods. Most commonly, the "response time" time is measured from the time the EMS receives the call to the arrival of EMS in the parking lot. Add another 1 to 2 minutes for PSAP dispatch, triage, and EMS notification, and another 1 to 2 minutes for EMS to actually get into your operatory, and the actual average "response time" is effectively 13 to 15 minutes from the time the OMS calls until a first responder is actually chairside. Fortunately, efforts are underway to standardize cardiac arrest response time statistics from "time of call" to "time of first shock."[16]

OPERATIONAL LOGISTICS OF EMERGENCY MEDICAL SERVICES SYSTEMS

The EMS system in the United States typically follows the Anglo-American model (bringing the patient to the hospital), as opposed to the Franco-German model (bringing the physician to the patient) of service delivery.[17] The majority of EMTs are employed by the municipal emergency service for their area, although this employer could itself be working under a number of models, including an autonomous public ambulance service, a fire department, a hospital-based service, or a private company working under contract.

In the United States, EMS providers give medical care under the authority and supervision of a medical director(s), usually an emergency physician who oversees the policies and protocols of a particular EMS system or organization, and the physician delegates that authority to EMS providers under his or her state's Medical Practice Act and Department of Health guidelines. The EMS activities and decisions may take place "on-line," where the EMS provider contacts the physician via phone or radio for direction or "off-line," where EMS personnel perform some or all procedures that follow standing medical orders. Under this paradigm, EMS personnel effectively assume the role of out-of-hospital field agents of hospital emergency physicians. Standing medical orders for any local are often openly shared when requested. This information would be of significant value to the OMS, who would then be able to anticipate the actions and roles of his or her local EMS.

THE FIRST RESPONDER CREDENTIALS

The credentials, training, and experience of the first responder can range from a policeman with minimal emergency skills and equipment, an EMT with limited basic life support (BLS) skills, to a paramedic with ALS skills and equipment. There are at least 40 types of certification of EMS personnel within the United States, and many of these are recognized by no more than a single state. The federal National Highway Transportation Safety Administration (NHTSA) has an EMS scope of practice model including minimum skills for various emergency responders.[18]

EMS qualification levels (per NHTSA guidelines) include (Appendix 1)[19]:

1. Emergency First Responder. The emergency first responder has completed a course in first aid, cardiopulmonary resuscitation, and AED use. The term "certified first responder" should not be confused with the generic term "first responder," referring to the first medically trained responder to arrive on scene (police, fire, or EMS). The primary focus of the emergency first responder is basic lifesaving care while awaiting additional EMS. If, as is often the case, the "first responder" is a policeman, realize that most in the United States are not trained in BLS, do not carry an AED, and, even if BLS trained, will often not perform BLS.[20]
2. Emergency Medical Technician—Basic (EMT-B). The EMT-B provides BLS and are limited to noninvasive procedures, such as

cardiopulmonary resuscitation, AED use, bag-valve-mask ventilation, placement of airway adjuncts (such as oral airways), pulse oximetry, and glucose testing using a glucometer. EMT-Bs are trained to assist patients with self-administration of prescribed medications, such as nitroglycerin, albuterol, and epineph-rine autoinjectors. Under the NHTSA curricu-lum, EMT-Bs undergo 110 hours of lecture and laboratory study.[17,19]

3. EMT—Intermediate (EMT-I). The intermediate medical technician provides limited advanced emergency medical care. The EMT-I is the new midlevel EMS provider introduced by the NHTSA according to the new EMS scope of practice model. The EMT-I scope consists of all EMT-B level skills, plus the insertion of supraglottic airways, suctioning of an already intubated patient, initiation of peripheral intra-venous therapy, including intravenous (IV) fluids, epinephrine, dextrose, glucagon, naloxone, and nitrous oxide. The EMT-I certifi-cation program is usually of 6 months duration, which includes clinical experience in operating rooms, emergency departments (EDs), and ALS ambulances.[17,19]

4. EMT-Paramedic. The paramedic provides advanced out-of-hospital emergency medical care, which generally includes some autono-mous functioning. In addition to all above EMT skills, the paramedic typically can perform endotracheal intubation and crico-thyrotomy, needle thoracotomy, gastric decompression, intraosseous cannula inser-tion, cardioversion, manual defibrillation, and transcutaneous pacing, and administer approved enteral and parenteral medications. In the United States, paramedic training is considered vocational, with program lengths from 1 to 2 years. EMT experience and certification are prerequisites, and most 2-year colleges offer an associate degree option.[17,19]

ROLES AND RESPONSIBILITIES DURING EMERGENCY MEDICAL SERVICES ARRIVAL

A staff member should meet EMS personnel at a prearranged office entrance, preferable one with direct access to the emergency and guide them to the site. Ensuing communication and events depend on the severity and urgency of the patient condition, the ability of the OMS to successfully provide or continue care and the ability and training of the responder. In certain situations, anxiety levels will be extremely high, which will hamper effective communication. Closed loop

communication and empowering team members to speak up is essential. It will be helpful to rely on mnemonics or acronyms such as the familiar "SOAP" note or "SBAR" (nursing hand-off), or the variation on SBAR used by EMS providers, SBAT.[21–24]

Situation/Scene: brief description of the inci-dent, patient's age, gender, problem;
Background: Previous medical history, medications;
Assessment: impression, stable versus unsta-ble, vital signs, electrocardiograph; and
Treatment/recommendation or request: treat-ment given and response, or a specific request.

During this or any emergency event/interven-tion, a staff member should be delegated to docu-ment all activities, to include:

1. The time of arrival of each EMS at the patient's side;
2. The names and titles of all EMS responders;
3. The time of the "hand-off" of the patient;
4. All interventions by EMS personnel;
5. The time the EMS leaves the office; and
6. The time the EMS leaves the parking lot.

EMS will also create their own incident report af-ter the intervention. Therefore, notes taken by the OMS team during the EMS response will be invalu-able documentation for the OMS.

ESTABLISHING AND MAINTAINING HIERARCHY WHEN EMERGENCY MEDICAL SERVICES IS ONSITE

It is entirely possible that EMS team(s) and OMS teams will be unknown to each other during the encounter despite advance preparation/rehearsal with local EMS personnel. Several different EMS providers, from different jurisdic-tions and with varied skill levels may gradually or eventually show up, which is a common sce-nario. In these situations, hand-off reports must be continually reiterated. The first to arrive can be a police officer, who may be unable or unwill-ing to assist. The second on the scene is most often a firefighter EMT, because firehouses are usually stationed nearby in strategic places throughout the community, and usually there are more firehouses than ambulance stations. In some cases, the last to arrive may be the one most needed: the EMT-paramedic, with ALS training and equipment. In the emergent sit-uation, the OMS will have to work with those pre-sent and quickly ascertain their scope of training, experience, and competence, which may not be obvious from their uniforms or insignia. Once confident in the skills of the EMS team, the OMS may decide to transfer care and responsibility.

To reiterate, the OMS can retain control of the patient while in his or her office until he or she is confident in the EMS capabilities and disposition of the patient. This act may require the OMS to contact the medical director of the EMS team to clarify the situation and assert control. The phone number of the local EMS medical director (eg, the ED direct line) should be part of your written office emergency protocol.

In the unfortunate possible event that various EMS providers and/or OMS cannot agree on treatment, will not communicate with each other, or will not coordinate as a team, as long as the patient is in the OMS office, the OMS has the right to continue to control the emergency treatment. Should the OMS wish to continue treatment control, and transport is necessary, then the OMS must accompany the patient during transport or cede control once the patient is outside of the office. EMS operates under the supervision of the physician in the ED and is directly responsible to that medical director and not the OMS. This situation may trigger discord, because the EMS may not take direction from the OMS, especially in instances where that recommended direction deviates from formal protocols. It is crucial to be mindful of the fact that, although EMS personnel may have more experience with ACLS and cardiac resuscitations, they will have only limited experience, at best, with anesthesia emergencies. In the event that the OMS retains control over the patient once EMS is on the scene, EMS may legally decline to work under the OMS supervision and will not provide treatment that does not comport with the EMS protocols. In particular, conflict may arise over methods of securing and maintaining the airway. For example, EMS providers are usually not familiar with laryngeal mask airways and may remove them on scene. Scenarios can take years to legally unfold; documentation is crucial.

EMERGENCY MEDICAL SERVICES TREATMENT AND TRANSPORT PROTOCOLS

There is ongoing controversy regarding the most effective way to use EMS resources. There are essentially 3 concepts, euphemistically called: "scoop and run," "stay and play," and "sweep and treat."[25] The stay and play concept espouses definitive treatment at the scene before transport and relies on improved EMS capabilities. This choice is not well-supported in the literature, and has been shown, in many cases to be detrimental to patient outcomes.[25–28]

The scoop and run concept is limited to immediate stabilization by EMS, followed by rapid transport to definitive care. It is generally believed by most medical directors that it is better to scoop and run than stay and play. However, current data relate only to the urban environment, where transport times to trauma centers are short. There may be more need for advanced techniques (ie, stay and play) in the rural environment or where transport times are prolonged. Stay and play is only useful if you cannot get the patient to a hospital in time without detrimental deterioration.[25–28]

Petrie and colleagues[28] report that, "even in large EMS systems, the median intubation rate is rarely more than 1 per year, with upward of 40% of practicing paramedics having performed none in any given 1-year period." Therefore, they ask, "Is it time to throw out intubation as a pre-hospital skill, given the realities of EMS practice?"

The final approach is sweep and treat, which means to perform most major interventions during transport. "There is ample experience . . . that for the very seriously injured, an en-route dedicated pre-hospital resuscitation . . . produced unexpected survivors."[25–28] In other words, transportation should not be delayed if stabilization can be accomplished en route: intubation, control of hemorrhage, medication delivery, and other services.

In summary, in an urban environment with relatively short transport times . . . there is no strong evidence supporting field ALS (by EMS) – and only a suggestion of harm. It is acknowledged that in very selected circumstances ALS maneuvers might be life-saving, but the rarity of such patients and the difficulty in maintaining competence if practiced only in these circumstances preclude any advantage at the population level to implementing pre-hospital ALS. During the design phase of a new trauma system in an urban setting, emphasis should be placed on efficient transport, on limited BLS interventions at the scene and on triage to a designated trauma center.[28]

THE HAND-OFF TO EMERGENCY MEDICAL SERVICES AND THE EMERGENCY DEPARTMENT

The EMS team will ask for a copy of your procedure and anesthesia record as a record of what transpired before they arrived to give to the ED. However, the

OMS' clinical record is a legal document that is the property of the OMS' office; the original should be retained by the OMS. You may be asked to make a copy of the clinical record, but it will almost certainly be incomplete at the time of transport, and may not accurately reflect transpired events. Tendered copies of medical records should be clearly marked as "INCOMPLETE RECORD." After the event, the OMS team should complete the record while it is still fresh in their memory and data are still available from the printout or memory of the vital signs monitor.

An OMS staff member should be delegated to record all events during EMS involvement and document those events on a separate emergency record form. This document will serve as a concise record of the event, giving the EMS team and the ED needed information. The emergency record, like the anesthesia record, should include vital signs every 5 minutes at a minimum, drugs given (doses and times), treatment given, response to interventions, and so on. It is recommended that a simple form for making quick notes be used during the actual emergency (Appendix 2), and afterward when there is time to recreate the event more thoroughly a more comprehensive form should be used (Appendix 3). Copies of these forms may be downloaded at http://www.fdsahome.org. These forms should also be marked as an "INCOMPLETE RECORD," then make a copy and give the copy to EMS to take to the ED.

The OMS should be informed of the name and location of the transport destination, and should call that facility to facilitate transfer of information and permit any preparation necessary by that facility. The SBAT format (Situation, Background, Assessment, Treatment/response) provides a concise report of the incident. Should the OMS elect to be present at the facility, this information can also be shared with health care providers.

POLICE AND EMERGENCY MEDICAL SERVICES

As discussed, the first responder at the scene may be a police officer, who will not be able to assist in the management of the emergency, but nonetheless may be in the office throughout the emergency. Ramifications of police presence include:

- Purposeful or inadvertent interference with the emergency response;
- Taking of records without permission;
- Refusal to allow OMS to leave the office and proceed to the ED; and
- Possible attempts to charge the OMS with "assault and battery."

Fortunately, these incidents are rare, but their rarity has left a void in the literature as to how to handle these situations. These issues seem to stem from the mistaken perception that the patient should not have suffered an emergency in a "dental" office undergoing a "dental" procedure and, therefore, by default the OMS must have done something wrong.

In general, the OMS does not have to permit the police into your office or provide them with records without a warrant. However, calling 911 generates a special situation, because you are for all intents and purposes inviting the police (as a first responder) into your office. Overall, remain calm, respectful, and compliant, and follow all instructions. The OMS's duty is to the care and treatment of the patient. If a police officer attempts to interfere with necessary resuscitation efforts the OMS should calmly remind the officer that the OMS is performing a life-saving procedure. If the police officer detains you, remind him that your presence is needed at the ED.

Rules in the Health Insurance Portability and Accountability Act of 1996 provide a wide variety of circumstances under which medical information can be disclosed for law enforcement–related purposes without explicitly requiring a warrant, one of which is in a medical emergency in connection with a crime. In other words, law enforcement is entitled to your records by simply asserting that you are now a suspect in a crime (ie, assault and battery) and they may take them from your office.[29]

IMPROVING THE EMERGENCY MEDICAL SERVICES–ORAL AND MAXILLOFACIAL SURGERY OFFICE INTERACTION

Given the problems that can occur with EMS in the OMS office, what can be done to understand how EMS works in your community, and to improve outcomes when EMS is activated? Effective teams practice and train together, but EMS crews often have revolving partners and rarely train with other provider teams, and EMS and OMS providers never train together, leading to potential medical errors. Highly functioning teams require effective leadership, group feedback, coordination of efforts, effective closed loop communication, and familiarity with tasks and individual roles, as described in advanced cardiac life support guidelines.

Regular office emergency simulation training can be used as an opportunity to get to know the local EMS team and to train together. Team simulation involving EMS can be requested and scheduled with your local EMS. In most cases, the EMS teams will be impressed with your initiative and happy to participate. Ideally, a high-fidelity

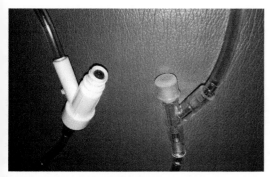

Fig. 1. Luer lock versus latex port.

SimMan simulator, an advanced cardiac life support or BLS mannequin, or at least an "airway management head" should be used for this exercise. Team simulation involving EMS then presents a great opportunity to inquire about the EMS systems, policies, response times, and protocols. An office tour can be arranged to share with them your emergency equipment and skills, and to ask for suggestions to improve your preparedness. Similarly, the medical director of your local EMS service (usually a physician at your local hospital ED) can be contacted to discuss their protocols or standing medical orders as they relate to the OMS office and EMS interface.

There are some specific EMS–OMS incompatibilities built into many OMS offices that should be considered. Most OMS offices are still using IV lines with latex injection ports, but the norm in medicine and EMS is to use Luer lock injection ports. This difference makes it difficult for EMS to use our IV lines in an emergency and may delay administration of emergency drugs. OMS offices should consider making the transition to all Luer lock IV lines (**Fig. 1**). Additionally, the OMS should be sure that preloaded emergency drugs come with both needles and Luer lock options (**Fig. 2**).

Performing chest compressions in a dental or surgery chair is unrealistic and ineffective. The chair is heavily padded and likely to rock under the pressure of compressions. OMS operatories are often too small to permit transferring the patient to the floor and still give complete team access to the patient. A team member should be prepared to slide a stool under the head of the surgery chair to stabilize the chair and to place a backboard under the patient (**Fig. 3**).

Small dental operatories (and even the typically larger OMS operatories) may make the EMS response difficult if the EMS team and all their equipment will not fit, so consideration should be given during the design of OMS operatories to make them large enough to accommodate an EMS team (**Fig. 4**). If the operatory is not large enough to fit the EMS gurney beside the dental chair, as is often the case, then the OMS should keep a patient transfer stretcher (such as the one shown in **Fig. 5**) in the office to facilitate transfer of the patient from the dental chair to the EMS gurney in the hallway.

GOOD SAMARITAN LAWS AND THE OFFICE EMERGENCY

Every state has a Good Samaritan law offering immunity to voluntary providers of emergency care, the specifics of which vary, but they do not apply when the emergency befalls a patient under active treatment in the office. They generally do apply to a bystander (eg, a family member in the waiting room) who suffers a medical emergency and the OMS team responds.[30]

There are generally several caveats for Good Samaritan protections to apply. First is that the injured victim must not object to the care offered or provided, but implied consent is assumed if the event is life threatening and the victim is unconscious. Second, the provider must act "reasonably and prudently." Stated another way, they do not apply if the provider acts in a "willful, wanton, or reckless manner." Third, the provider must not act in the hope of being paid or rewarded.[30]

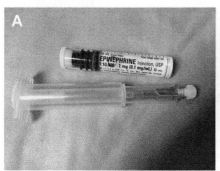
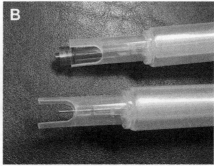

Fig. 2. (*A*) Luer lock and needle syringe. (*B*) Luer lock versus needle syringe.

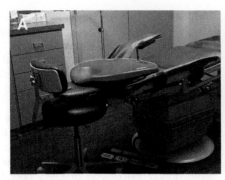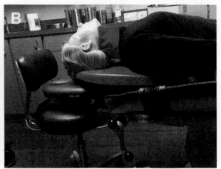

Fig. 3. (*A*) Cardiopulmonary resuscitation (CPR) setup for surgery chair. (*B*) CPR setup for surgery chair.

Florida's Good Samaritan Act is a representative example of state statutes[31]:

Florida Statute 768.13 Good Samaritan Act; immunity from civil liability. —

> *(2) (a) Any person, including those licensed to practice medicine, ... who ... in good faith renders emergency care or treatment either in direct response to emergency ... outside of a hospital, doctor's office, or other place having proper medical equipment, without objection of the injured victim or victims thereof, shall not be held liable for any civil damages as a result of such care or treatment or as a result of any act or failure to ... where the person acts as an ordinary reasonably prudent person would have acted under the same or similar circumstances.*

Additionally, be aware that most states require written notification of the state Dental Board within 48 hours of any emergency requiring the transfer of a patient to the ED.

> Florida Administrative Code, Rule 64B5-14.006 Reporting of Adverse Occurrences[32]

> *1. Definition:*
> *a. Adverse occurrence - ... an incident that . . . requires hospitalization or emergency room treatment of a dental patient.*
> *2. Any dentist practicing in the state of Florida must notify the Board in writing by registered mail within 48 hours of any . . . adverse occurrence that occurs in the dentist's outpatient facility.*

The board notification requirement should never deter an OMS from requesting emergency assistance from EMS; state boards generally understand that getting emergency assistance is always the better decision and is not an admission of error on the part of the dentist.

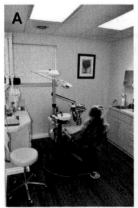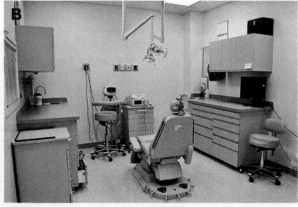

Fig. 4. (*A*) Cardiopulmonary resuscitation (CPR) set-up for surgery chair. (*B*) Larger oral and maxillofacial surgery operatory. (*Data from* [*A*] 2017. Available at: https://pxhere.com/en/photo/569155; and Available at: https://creativecommons.org/publicdomain/zero/1.0/. Accessed July 25, 2017; and [*B*] License: CC0 Public Domain. Available at: https://www.baypines.va.gov/BAYPINES/clinemp/DentalCareer/1Benefits.asp. Accessed July 31, 2017.

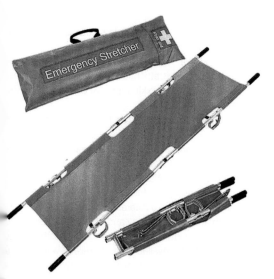

Fig. 5. Folding transfer stretcher.

SUMMARY

The OMS should expect that what can happen, will happen eventually. But due to the rarity of medical emergencies, the OMS will undoubtedly have an inherent response conflict ranging from, "I can't believe this is happening," and "I have no experience," to "first do no harm." But patients generally do better when you act, than when you do not. Remember Campbell's Law: "In an emergency, an act of omission is usually worse than an act of commission" (Robert L. Campbell, DDS, oral communication, February 2017). In other words, do not let the fear of making a mistake cause you to freeze and do nothing. Generally err on side of aggressive treatment. Empower your staff to act and communicate. There are many documented malpractice cases where EMS arrived and found the dental team standing around doing nothing (or not enough) while they wait for EMS, and by then it is usually too late.

It should be obvious from this discussion that there is more to activating EMS than just telling a staff member to "call 911" and that forethought, planning, documentation, and team simulation training must be undertaken to make it effective.

EMS is not definitive care, the ED is, and that is where the patient needs to be a soon as possible. Do not count on EMS to arrive and "save the day." The office-based OMS providing office-based anesthesia must be proactive and call early in an emergency, and must be prepared to stabilize and maintain the patient for at least 15 minutes.

REFERENCES

1. 911 and E911 Services. Federal Communications Commission. 2017. Available at: https://www.fcc.gov/general/9-1-1-and-e9-1-1-services. Accessed July 24, 2017.
2. 9-1-1 Origin & History. National Emergency Number Association Website. Available at: http://www.nena.org/?page=911overviewfacts. Accessed July 24, 2017.
3. Next-Generation 9-1-1. Intelligent Transportation Systems Joint Program Office. Available at: https://www.its.dot.gov/research_archives/ng911/index.htm. Accessed July 24, 2017.
4. Malamed SF. Basic principles and resuscitation. Chapter 1. In: Dolan J, editor. Medical emergencies in the dental office. 6th edition. St Louis (MO): Mosby; 2007. p. 59–65.
5. Hass DA. Preparing dental office staff members for emergencies. J Am Dental Assoc 2010;141:8–13.
6. Bennett JD, Rosenberg MB. Medical emergencies in dentistry. Philadelphia: Saunders; 2002.
7. Kaltman S, Ragan M, Borges O. Managing the untoward anesthetic event in an OMS practice. Oral Maxillofacial Surg Clin North Am 2013;25(3):515–27.
8. Peikoff K. CPR survival rates can differ greatly by city. The New York Times 2015. Available at: https://www.nytimes.com/2015/12/08/health/cpr-survival-rates-can-differ-greatly-by-city.html. Accessed July 24, 2017.
9. 46-fold difference in cardiac arrest survival. University of Washington. Available at: https://depts.washington.edu/survive/46fold.php. Accessed July 24, 2017.
10. Fitch J. Response times: myths, measurement and management. J Emerg Med 2005;30(9):47–56. Available at: http://www.jems.com/articles/2005/08/response-times-myths44-measure.html. Accessed July 31, 2017.
11. National Fire Prevention Association. NFPA 1710, Standard for the Organization and Deployment of Fire Suppression Operations, Emergency Medical Operations, and Special Operations to the Public by Career Fire Departments. Quincy (MA): National Fire Prevention Association; 2016. Available at: http://www.nfpa.org/codes-and-standards/all-codes-and-standards/list-of-codes-and-standards/detail?code=1710.
12. EMS Response Time Standards. EMS World 2004. Available at: http://www.emsworld.com/article/10324786/ems-response-time-standards. Accessed July 24, 2017.
13. Emergency Medical Services Performance Measures. National Highway Traffic Safety Administration. 2009. Available at: https://www.ems.gov/pdf/811211.pdf. Accessed July 24, 2017.

14. USA today series examines disparities in emergency medical services. Kaiser Health News 2009. Available at: http://khn.org/morning-breakout/dr00019077/. Accessed July 24, 2017.

15. Many lives are lost across USA because emergency services fail. USA Today 2005. Available at: http://usatoday30.usatoday.com/news/nation/ems-day1-cover.htm. Accessed July 24, 2017.

16. Institute of Medicine. Board on Health Sciences Policy, Committee on the Treatment of Cardiac Arrest: Current Status and Future Directions. Emergency medical services response to cardiac arrest. In: Graham R, McCoy MA, Schultz AM, editors. Strategies to improve cardiac arrest survival: a time to act. Washington, DC: The National Academies Press; 2015.

17. Dick WF. Anglo-American vs. Franco-German Emergency medical services system. Prehosp Disaster Med 2003;18(1):29–37.

18. National EMS Scope of Practice Medicine. EMS.gov. 2007. Available at: https://www.ems.gov/education/EMSScope.pdf. Accessed July 24, 2017.

19. National Emergency Medical Services Education Standards. EMS.gov. 2009. Available at: https://www.ems.gov/pdf/education/National-EMS-Education-Standards-and-Instructional-Guidelines/EMR_Instructional_Guidelines.pdf. Accessed July 24, 2017.

20. Brody J. Increasing CPR training to save lives. New York Times 2016. Available at: https://www.nytimes.com/2016/10/25/well/live/increasing-cpr-training-to-save-people-in-cardiac-arrest.html. Accessed July 24, 2017.

21. Wurster FW. Mnemonic device helps patient hand-offs. J Emerg Med Serv 2011;36(7):32–4. Available at: http://www.jems.com/articles/print/volume-36/issue-7/training/mnemonic-device-helps-patient-hand-offs.html. Accessed July 25, 2017.

22. Wurster FW. The hand-off: smooth transitions between healthcare providers. JEMS 2011;36(7) 32, 34.

23. SBAR Toolkit. Institute for Healthcare Improvement. Available at: http://www.ihi.org/resources/Pages/Tools/sbartoolkit.aspx. Accessed July 25, 2017.

24. Duckworth RL. Five ways to perfect the patient handoff. EMS World 2016. Available at: http://www.emsworld.com/article/12257122/five-ways-to-perfect-the-patient-handoff. Accessed July 25, 2017.

25. Smith RM, Conn AK. Prehospital care - scoop and run or stay and play? Injury 2009;40(Suppl 4):S23–6.

26. Bleecher C. Are there differences in outcomes between "scoop and run" and "stay and play" pre-hospital care models? San Francisco (CA): Trauma Anesthesiology Society; 2016. Available at: https://www.tashq.org, are-there-differences-in-outcomes-between-scoop-and-run-and-stay-and-play-pre-hospital-care-models/. Accessed July 25, 2017.

27. Haas B, Nathens AB. Pro/con debate: is the scoop and run approach the best approach to trauma services organization? Crit Care 2008;12: 224.

28. Petrie D, Tallon J, Kovacs G. Pre-hospital airway management: the evidence. Chapter 21. In: Malley J, editor. Airway management in emergencies. Shelton (CT): Peoples Medical Publishing House USA Ltd (PMPH); 2011. p. 403–8.

29. FAQ on Government Access to Medical Records. American Civil Liberties Union. Available at: https://www.aclu.org/other/faq-government-access-medical-records. Accessed July 26, 2017.

30. Judson K, Harrison C. Law and ethics for the health professions. 7th edition. New York: McGraw Hill; 2016. p. 188–9.

31. Fla. Stat. §768.13.

32. Fla. Admin. Code Rule §64B5–14.006.

APPENDIX 1: SKILL SETS FOR VARIOUS LEVELS OF EMS PROVIDER

Emergency Medical Responder	Emergency Medical Technician	Advanced EMT	Paramedic
EMS provider airway and breathing skill set			
Oral airway BVM Sellick's maneuver Head-tilt chin lift jaw-thrust Modified chin lift obstruction–manual Nasal cannula oxygen Nonrebreather face mask Upper airway suctioning	Humidifiers Partial rebreathers Venturi mask, manually triggered ventilator Oral and nasal airways	Combitube, King airways	BiPAP/CPAP Needle chest decompression Chest tube monitoring Cricothyrotomy NG/OG tube Endotracheal intubation Airway obstruction removal by direct laryngoscopy PEEP
EMS provider assessment skill Set			
Manual BP	Pulse oximetry Manual and auto BP	Blood glucose monitor	ECG interpretation interpretive 12 Lead Blood chemistry analysis Capnography
EMS provider cardiac skill set			
CPR AED	Mechanical CPR		Cardioversion Carotid massage Manual defibrillation TC pacing
EMS provider pharmacologic skill set			
Assisted medication • Unit dose autoinjectors for self-care	Assisted medications • Assisting a patient in administering their own prescribed medications, including autoinjection Tech of Med administration • Buccal • Oral Administered Meds • OTC medications (glucose, ASA for chest pain of suspected ischemic origin)	Peripheral IV insertion IV fluid infusion Pediatric IO Tech of Med Administration • Aerosolized • Subcutaneous • Intramuscular • Nebulized • Sublingual • Intranasal • IV push D50, Narcan Administered Meds • SL nitroglycerine • SQ or IM epinephrine • Glucagon and IV D50 • Inhaled beta agonist • Narcotic antagonist • Nitrous oxide for pain relief	Central line monitoring IO insertion Venous blood sampling Tech of Med Administration • Endotracheal • IV (push and infusion) • NG • Rectal • IO • Topical • Accessing implanted central IV port Administered Meds • Physician-approved medications • Maintenance of blood administration • Thrombolytics initiation

Abbreviations: AED, automated external defibrillator; ASA, aspirin; BiPAP, biphasic positive airways pressure; BP, blood pressure; BVM, bag-valve-mask; CPAP, continuous positive airway pressure; CPR, cardiopulmonary resuscitation; ECG, electrocardiograph; EMS, emergency medical services; EMT, emergency medical technician; IM, intramuscular; IO, intraosseous; IV, intravenous; NG/OG, nasogastric/orogastric; OTC, over the counter; PEEP, positive end-expiratory pressure; SL, sublingual; SQ, subcutaneous; TC, transcutaneous.

From National Highway Traffic Safety Administration. National EMS scope of practice model. 2007. Available at: https://www.ems.gov/education/EMSScope.pdf. Accessed July 24, 2017.

APPENDIX 2: SIMPLE MEDICAL EMERGENCY RECORD FORM

Medical Emergency Record

BVM – bag valve mask
PPV – positive pressure ventilation
OPA – oropharyngeal airway placed
SUX – succinylcholine, IV
iGEL – iGEL supraglottic airway
ETT - Intubate
End Tidal CO_2
REMEMBER:
Epi 1:1,000 = IM
Epi 1:10,000 = IV

Time of 911 call_____ Time of EMS arrival_____

EMS status: ____police ____EMT ____paramedic _ ___unidentified

PATIENT NAME _____Date_____   ◯ IF APPLIES

Awake, Breathing, Talking

TIME	STATUS / INTERVENTION	Vital Signs (BP, HR SpO₂,CO₂ waveform?)	
0935	e.g. Lost airway, Triple airway, suction	e.g. 120/80 ;65; 95%; Yes (No)	A B T
0937	BVM with PPV @ 15 lpm O₂	92%; Yes (No)	A B T
0939	iGel placed	139/92; 93; 99%; (Yes) No	A B T
0940	Narcan 1ml given IV	(Yes) No	(A)(B) T
		Yes No	A B T
		Yes No	A B T
		Yes No	A B T
		Yes No	A B T
		Yes No	A B T

Courtesy of Robert C. Bosack, DDS, Orland Park, IL.

APPENDIX 3: COMPLETE MEDICAL EMERGENCY RECORD FORM

MEDICAL EMERGENCY RECORD
(Time line, sympts, Dx, airway, 0₂, IV, meds./CPR)
Time (1 large block = 5 mins; 1 small block = 1 min)

Patient Name: _____ Date: _____
Diagnosis: _____ Time: _____ 911 Call Time _____

Vital Signs	Pulse									
	Systolic BP									
	Diastolic BP									
	Pulse Oximeter									
	Pulse - Reg. Or Irreg.									

Signs/Sympts./Events: table at right & bk of form for add. details
Diagnosis: enter #, and place # next to EMERGENCY below

EMERGENCY:	Drug:									Total Dose
For any emergency	IV Fluids: NS, LR, Other:									
	Oxygen - L/min.									
	Airway Management:									
Acute Adrenal Insufficiency	Hydrocort./Dexameth.– mg IV									
ACS - Angina Pectoris	Nitroglyc. - spray / tab (sublingual)									
ACS - Myocardial Infarction	Morphine Sulfate - mg IV									
	Aspirin - mg po (tablet)									
Allergic Reaction:	Epineph. 1:1000 - mg IM									
• Mild	Benadryl - mg IV									
• Severe	Decadron - mg IV									
• Anaphylaxis	Ranitidine - mg IV									
Bronchospasm / Asthma	Albuterol - puff (metered dose)									
	Epi. - mg 1:1000 IM / 1:10,000 IV									
CARDIAC DYSRHYTHMIAS										
• Bradycardia (symptomatic)	Atropine - mg IV									
	Epinephrine - mcg / min									
• Tachy.- Nar., Reg.(SVT)	Adenosine - mg IV									
• Tachy.- Nar., Irreg.	Diltiazem - mg IV									
	Metoprolol - mg IV									
• Tachy. - Wide, VT	Amiodarone - mg IV									
	Procainamide - mg IV									
	Adenosine - mg IV									
• Tachy. - Wide, VT Torsades	Mag. Sulfate – mg IV									
• Ectopy – Significant: UF, MF	Lidocaine – mg IV; mg / min									
Cardiac Dysrhytmias – Pulseless Arrest Rhythms										
• VF / VT (pulseless)	Epinephrine (1:10,000) - mg IV(E)									
	Amiodarone - mg IV(A)									
C,D;C(IV),D;C(E),D;C(A),D;	Lidocaine - mg IV									
Repeat C(E),D;C(A),D	CPR (C) / Defib. (D)									
• Asystole / PEA	Epinephrine (1:10,000) - mg IV									
	CPR (C) / Defib. (D)									

 # SIGN/SYMPTOM

APPEARANCE
Di = Diaphoresis
T = Tearing
Sw = Swelling; eye, lip, tongue
Pa = Pallor
Cy = Cyanosis

SKIN/SOFT TISS.
P = Pruritus
R = Rash
H = Hives
E = Erythema

NEUROLOGIC
A = Anxiety
CN = Confusion
Wk = Weakness
LC = Loss consc.

CARDIOVASCULAR
CP = Chest Pain
Br = Brady
Tk = Tachy
Thr = Thready
Plp = Palpitations
NP = No pulse

RESPIRATORY
Cr = Crowing
SR = Supra-sternal retraction
NE = No exchange
RV = Resist.Vent.
Wh = Wheezing
Cgh = Cough
G = Gasping
S = Stridor
Dy = Dyspnea
Hp = Hypopnea
A = Apnea

MUSCULOSKELETAL
Ms = Musc. spsm
Fl = Flail
Wk = Weakness
R = Rigid

GASTROINTESTINAL
N = Nausea
V = Vomiting

AIRWAY ADJUNCTS
N = Nasal Mask
F = Face Mask
C = Cannula
NA = Nasal AW
OA = Oral AW
E = ET
L = LMA
I = Igel
IA = Inhal. Adptr.
Cr = Cricothyrot.

• Total • Dose

Time (1 block = 5 min., 1 dot = 1 min.)

Emesis & Aspiration	Succinylcholine – mg IV (intub.)									
	Rocuronium – mg IV (intub.)									
	Sugammadex – mg IV									
Hyperventilation	Midazolam - mg IV									
Hypertension	Labetalol - mg IV									
	Esmolol - mg IV / mcg/kg/min									
	Hydralazine - mg IV									
Hypoglycemia - Insulin Shock	Glucose p.o. – packets / juice									
	Dextrose - mg IV									
	Glucagon - mg IM									
Hypotension	Ephedrine - mg IV									
	Phenylephrine – mg IV									
	Vasopressin 20u/L– ml/min.									
Intra-arterial Injection	Lidocaine 1% (w/o epi) - ml IV									
Laryngospasm	Succinylcholine - mg IV									
	Rocuronium - mg IV									
	Sugammadex – mg IV									
Respiratory Depression	Naloxone (Narcotic) - mg IV									
	Flumazenil (BZDP) - mg IV									
Syncope	Ammonia - inhalant vial									
	Atropine – mg IV									
Seizure	Midazolam - mg IV / IM / buccal									
	Valium - mg IV									

TIME:	EVENTS / SYMPTOMS / NON-PHARMOCOLOGIC INTERVENTIONS / COMMENTS:

EMERGENCY STAFF/ DISCHARGE

Assist. #1:	Assist. #3:	Aux. Desk #1
Assist. #2:	Assist. #4	Aux. Desk #2:
Patient discharged to:		Time:
Discharge Condition:		

Courtesy of Richard C. Robert, DDS, San Francisco, CA.

Preoperative Evaluation and Patient Selection for Office-Based Oral Surgery Anesthesia

Stuart Lieblich, DMD[a,b,*]

KEYWORDS

- Preoperative assessment • METs • Systemic diseases

KEY POINTS

- Patient evaluation for risk determination is vital to reduce adverse events.
- A focused physical examination including baseline vital signs should be part of the patient evaluation.
- Modification of anesthetic techniques may be necessary based on preexisting comorbidities.
- Routine laboratory tests are not indicated, but specific testing based on medical conditions may be indicated.

The oral and maxillofacial surgeon (OMS) care of the patient starts with an initial evaluation of the patient's medical history. The goal is to ascertain whether the patient can tolerate the insult of the surgical procedure as well as the anesthetic technique. Because this issue deals with anesthetic issues, medical conditions that potentially affect patient outcomes are also reviewed.

As the OMS evaluates the patient, consideration of the individual's reserve and resiliency needs to be ascertained. Although similar in concept, the patient's ability to maintain homeostasis through potentially adverse events (hypoxia, hypercarbia, fluid shifts) needs to be determined before the anesthetic. Therefore, patient evaluation starts with a thorough medical history and includes questions about previous surgical and anesthetic experiences. This article guides the clinician through a systematic review of the patient's health status in preparation for an office anesthetic. It will be obvious as well to the reader that there are no specific algorithms that can precisely determine an individual's risk of an adverse event during an anesthetic. The professional judgment of the practitioner is always the primary determinant and does not supersede any of the information discussed later.

Many risk assessment tools used in the hospital operating room setting are not directly applicable to the OMS practice because, although the planned surgeries are in the maxillofacial region, acute issues of blood loss and fluid shifts are not expected. However, the issues of working in an open and unsecured airway are important considerations and somewhat unique in the OMS practice.

GENERAL PATIENT EVALUATION

The ideal situation in an office practice is to have an initial consultation with a patient at an appointment that precedes the surgical date. This initial consultation allows the OMS time to fully evaluate a patient, to obtain any additional laboratory studies or information, and perhaps

[a] University of Connecticut School of Dental Medicine, Farmington, CT, USA; [b] Private Practice, Avon Oral and Maxillofacial Surgery, 34 Dale Road, Suite 105, Avon, CT 06001, USA
* Corresponding author. Private Practice, Avon Oral and Maxillofacial Surgery, 34 Dale Road, Suite 105, Avon, CT 06001.
E-mail address: StuL@comcast.net

Oral Maxillofacial Surg Clin N Am 30 (2018) 137–144
https://doi.org/10.1016/j.coms.2018.01.001
1042-3699/18/© 2018 Elsevier Inc. All rights reserved.

to modify the patient's pharmacologic regimen before the surgery. It also allows the OMS to plan an appropriate anesthetic in consultation with the patient's needs. It is well understood that many procedures can be accomplished with just a local anesthetic, and there are situations in which the patient may not tolerate that option.

As the OMS is typically initially meeting the patient for the first time, it is ideal if patients can complete their medical history forms at home before presenting to the office. Pre-completion may permit the patient more time to gather the information before the consultation, perhaps with discussion with another family member. If submitted ahead of time electronically to the office, the staff may have time to perform an initial review of the patient's medical history. Certainly, accuracy and completeness may be enhanced if done outside of the office setting.

Baseline vital signs are obtained at the patient's visit. Baseline vital signs include recording of the blood pressure and pulse rate/rhythm. Many offices will initially place the noninvasive blood pressure and pulse oximeter during the initial intake of a patient. If delegated to a staff member, training in the recognition of abnormal rhythms must be done for this to be valuable. Staff should understand and recognize common arrhythmias, such as the irregularly irregular rhythm of atrial fibrillation (AF) by palpation or the audible sound of the pulse oximeter and alert the OMS of its presence. These values should be recorded on the patient's record at this visit as well. If the practice's electronic medical record does not flag abnormal values, the doctor should be alerted to any values outside a set parameter (eg, blood pressures >150/90 mm Hg).

The next step is for the OMS to review the patient's past medical and surgical history. As information is gathered, assignment of the patient's American Society of Anesthesiologists (ASA) physical status is determined and recorded in the patient's medical history. The ASA status provides documentation that the OMS has indeed reviewed the patient's list of medical conditions and assessed the level of control of these conditions. Past surgical procedures should be discussed with the patient to ascertain how they tolerated the anesthetic. Often patients may reply that they have reactions to anesthetics or certain medications when in fact they are mostly side effects, such as nausea and vomiting. However, issues such as delayed awakening from an anesthetic or respiratory complications may alert the OMS that additional details are necessary.

CHECKLIST FOR PATIENT EVALUATION FOR AN OFFICE ANESTHETIC

1. Blood pressure
2. Heart rate and rhythm
3. Past medical history, reviewed and verified
4. Current medications, including recent changes in medications
5. Risk factor evaluation for sleep apnea
6. Past surgical history and responses to anesthesia, family history review of anesthetic complications
7. Salient laboratory result review
   a. Electrocardiogram (ECG) for patients with cardiac disease (within 6–12 months)
   b. Blood glucose levels and $HgBA_{1c}$ for diabetics (type I and type II)
   c. International normalized ratio (INR) reports for patients taking warfarin (within 7 days of planned surgery) or suspected hepatic disease
   d. Spo_2 on room air for patients with respiratory disease
8. Recording of metabolic equivalent (MET) functional capacity
9. Recording of ASA status

PATIENT PHYSICAL EXAMINATION FOR AN OFFICE ANESTHETIC

1. Focused airway examination
   a. Mallampati score recorded
   b. Range of opening
   c. Risk factors predicting difficulty with positive pressure ventilation
2. Auscultation of lungs
3. Observation of extremities for venipuncture sites

Contemporary preanesthetic evaluation has for the most part eliminated the need for routine laboratory testing. Instead, the above patient screening results will alert the practitioner about the possibility of an undiagnosed or undertreated medical condition. The role of the OMS is not to be the patient's primary care physician. However, one must remain vigilant to the possibility that the patient's medical condition may be insidiously exacerbating without a specific alerting sign to the patient. Significant information can be obtained by determining the patient's MET level. In this author's opinion, it offers the best insight into a patient's ability to withstand an adverse anesthetic event. The functional status assessment (MET) level is based on assigning the value of 1 to the amount of oxygen consumption at rest in a chair (**Table 1**). Each increase is an increment of that so an MET level of 4 is activity that uses

Table 1
Functional status assessment (metabolic equivalent task) examples

Excellent (>7 METs)	Moderate (4–7 METs)	Poor (<4 METs)
Squash, jogging (10-min mile), scrubbing floors, singles tennis	Cycling, climbing a flight of stairs, golf (without cart), walking 4 mph, yard work (eg, raking leaves, weeding, pushing a power mower)	Vacuuming, activities of daily living (eg, eating, dressing, bathing), walking 2 mph, writing

Data from Hlatky MA, Boineau RE, Higginbotham MB, et al. A brief self-administered questionnaire to determine functional capacity (the Duke Activity Status Index). Am J Cardiol 1989;64:651–4.

times the oxygen consumption than at rest. This nonconfrontational evaluation can provide significant information regarding the patient's cardiac and respiratory reserve. The astute clinician may pick up on changes in the patient's responses. For example, they may report, "I used to walk the golf course but now I regularly take a golf cart." This statement may indicate that there is slow decline in this individual's respiratory or cardiac reserve that they are even unaware of. Positive findings of a level of 4 METs or less would indicate the patient is not optimal for an office anesthetic because of their lack of cardiac and/or respiratory reserve.

One exception to the indication for routine laboratory testing may be female patients of child-bearing age. The American Association of Oral and Maxillofacial Surgeons' Parameters of Care does not endorse routine testing for pregnancy.[1] Exceptions may be indicated if there is an equivocal history of sexual activity with a possibility of pregnancy because of an uncertainty regarding the time of the last menstrual period. Because there are concerns about the teratogenic effects of some anesthetic medications and the potential harm to the developing fetus, this discussion should be noted in the patient's record. A urine testing kit for pregnancy is usually positive within 14 days of conception (blood tests will be positive in 10 days) and that option can be offered to a patient (Shlansky L, personal communication, 2018) with an equivocal history.

SPECIFIC PATIENT EVALUATION ISSUES
Cardiac Disease

A patient with a history of cardiac disease will appropriately raise the level of concern of the OMS and consideration of further evaluation of the individual's status. Good historians can often provide adequate information about their status to allow the OMS to determine if further information and tests are needed. Certainly, consideration for consultation with the patient's cardiologist may be indicated especially if the cardiac event was recent. For example, a patient with a history of a myocardial infarction (MI) will require a determination of the severity of the cardiac insult. Because cardiac muscle does not "heal" after an infarction, understanding the severity of the MI should be determined. Here too a discussion of the patient's medications, and especially any changes in medications, will give some insights. The OMS should inquire about the individual's MET level and again if there has been any decline over the past few months. Recent risk assessment studies show that chance of a second MI stabilizes by 3 months following the initial event but of course remains significantly higher than an individual that never had an MI. More "urgent" procedures can be considered as soon as 1 month following an MI, but here too cardiology consultation should be involved.

Cardiac arrhythmias, particularly AF, should be investigated. The office staff may detect the irregularity on initial obtaining of vital signs. In addition, the use of medications such as warfarin or other direct-acting oral anticoagulants (DOACs) may provide this insight even in patients who do not report it on their medical history. Concerns about patients in chronic AF relate to tachycardias, which can lead to acute decompensation and heart failure. Certainly, the anesthetic plan should limit that possibility (avoiding anticholinergics such as atropine; limiting/avoiding the use of epinephrine; and judicious fluid replacement). Patients with chronic AF and a rate greater than 90 bpm should be considered for cardiology referral to achieve optimal rate control.

Consideration of obtaining a recent ECG report in patients with cardiac disease and having a dialogue with the cardiologist may improve risk assessment in this population. Because many of these patients are on various anticoagulants, a discussion about the possibility of discontinuing can also be held. Certainly, many studies show that with an INR of less than 4, warfarin can be continued and local measures used for hemostasis. However, there is no laboratory test for the effects of DOACs, and consideration for cessation is based on the risks of bleeding versus the risk of clot formation with holding these drugs. The OMS will need to communicate the risks of postoperative bleeding to the cardiologist. For example, following dental extractions, direct measures to permit hemostasis can readily be used even if postextraction oozing occurs. In contrast, bleeding into an open space such as the maxillary sinus or the floor of the mouth may be associated with higher morbidity and difficulty in control.

The preoperative evaluation of patients with implanted pacemakers and internal defibrillators (ICDs) usually warrants cardiac consultation. The electrical spike of the pacemaker can be detected on the ECG in lead II. If the patient has a demand pacemaker that only spikes when the rate drops below a certain point, a spike may not be seen with an adequate spontaneous rhythm. These patients are inherently more stable and may have a better cardiac response to hemodynamic changes under anesthesia. ICDs can cardiovert ventricular tachycardia and defibrillate ventricular fibrillation. In contrast, these patients can be assumed to have a more fragile cardiac condition and may not tolerate the stress of even treatment with local anesthetics alone.

Congestive heart failure is a progressive loss of the normal cardiac output. Presenting symptoms of uncompensated heart failure include shortness of breath and increasing fatigue. Right-sided failure may present with pulmonary symptoms due to pulmonary congestion, and left-sided failure may present with peripheral edema, although isolated left- or right-sided failure is not typically seen. Here again, the evaluation of the patient's MET level and especially reduction in MET level may indicate worsening of the patient's disease. These individuals cannot tolerate acute changes in heart rate or blood pressure, and the anesthetic plan might include monitoring of the patient's blood pressure and lead II ECG even if treatment with just local anesthesia is considered.

Respiratory Disease

One of the major risks of an office anesthetic delivered via an open airway is the development of apnea/hypopnea due to the anesthetic medications. The improvement in monitoring with pulse oximetry and end tidal carbon dioxide will alert the OMS that the situation is occurring, permitting intervention. The amount of time the OMS has before significant hypoxemia and hypercarbia occur will be based on the respiratory status of the patient. Understanding that the healthy 70-kg adult has a much greater pulmonary reserve than a morbidly obese individual illustrates that intervention must be more rapid and efficient in the compromised patient (**Fig. 1**).

Probably the most common chronic respiratory disease that the OMS will encounter is asthma. The asthmatic patient needs specific evaluation as to the severity of their disease. A report of exercise-induced asthma exacerbation ("attack") that rapidly responds to a beta-2 agonist agent (eg, albuterol) can typically be safely treated in the office setting. Consideration of pretreatment with an inhaler is often mentioned as adjunctive therapy just before an anesthetic. Because there are minimal cardiac effects with these agents, there is little risk to its use; however, no benefits

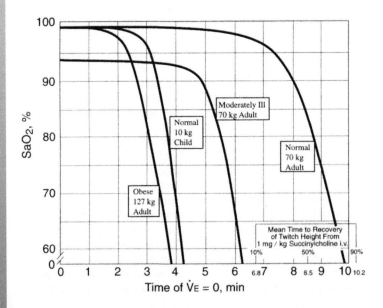

Fig. 1. Time to hemoglobin desaturation with initial $F_AO_2 = 0.87$. (*From* Benumof JF, Dagg R, Benumof R. Critical hemoglobin desaturation will occur before return to an unparalyzed state following 1 mg/kg intravenous succinylcholine. Anesthesiology 1997;87(4):980; with permission.)

have been shown for prophylactic use in patients without wheezing. Auscultation of the lungs of the asthmatic should be undertaken before an anesthetic to rule out any preoperative wheezing.

More moderate to severe asthmatics will be on a regimen of a daily inhaled corticosteroid with the need for rescue inhalers as well as occasional need for oral corticosteroids or emergency department visits. Although many asthmatics may be aware of their specific triggers and can usually avoid them, the psychological stress of surgery may cause an acute exacerbation.

Consideration for avoidance of known releasers of histamine such as meperidine is often mentioned in the context of asthmatics, although this author has not found this to be an issue with mild asthmatics. The sympathomimetic effects of ketamine are also mentioned as potentially an adjunct because of its bronchodilation effects. However, the increased secretions may predispose patients to upper respiratory embarrassment (eg, laryngospasm) so its use in this group of patients may not be as useful.

In the context of asthma, there is also significant discussion in the anesthesia literature regarding the management of a patient with a recent history of an upper respiratory infection (URI). Many have recommended deferral of an anesthetic for at least 4 weeks following a URI. Although some studies do indeed show an increase in postanesthetic respiratory adverse events (PRADEs), in these patients the primary risk is involved with endotracheal intubation, causing stimulation to the reactive airway. In contrast, mask anesthetics in children without signs of an acute URI (mucopurulent secretions, fever, lethargy, and lower respiratory congestion) are not associated with an increase in PRADEs.[2]

Cigarette smoking may cause a reduction in oxygen reserve because of the binding of carbon monoxide to hemoglobin. Ideally, patients should stop smoking at least 24 hours before an anesthetic to reduce the concentration of carbon monoxide. Some references however note an increased mucous production with smoking cessation, and this may predispose the patient to laryngospasm or other airway issues. A meta-analysis of studies[3] seems to indicate that reduction in respiratory complications after anesthesia only occurs with at least 4 weeks of cessation. Less than that has no effect on outcomes. The correlation of this information to the OMS model of anesthesia has not been studied. Therefore, the smoker should be evaluated in terms of their respiratory capacity, and here an MET level of greater than 4 should not be associated with an increased risk for an office anesthetic.

Hepatic Disease

There are various causes of hepatic disease, including viral hepatitis, chronic alcoholism, and damage from other drugs (acetaminophen). The specific cause of the disease is not particularly relevant to the patient evaluation, but assessing the degree of hepatic function is.

A patient with hepatic disease may not present with any specific anesthetic risks, per se. Usually 80% to 90% of the liver cells (hepatocytes) must be nonfunctional for the clinical signs of hepatic failure to become noticeable. However, as hepatic disease progresses, various homeostatic aspects become compromised, especially the reduction of albumin and other plasma proteins. Appreciating that most anesthetic drugs are highly protein bound (benzodiazepines, local anesthetics), a reduction in these proteins creates a greater amount of free drug in the central circulation. Toxic levels of local anesthetics can occur more readily, and delayed recovery from an anesthetic may also be noted.[4] Decreased hepatic enzymes can lead to delayed metabolism and subsequent excretion of drugs. Decreased hepatic function may not be clinically relevant given that recovery from an office anesthetic is associated with redistribution of drugs, not metabolism or elimination. The role for rapidly redistributed drugs such as propofol versus benzodiazepines may be recommended in these patients.

Because the liver is also responsible for production of clotting agents (with the exception of factor VIII), the risk of postoperative bleeding may occur. If the INR is elevated greater than 1.5, a significant amount of hepatic failure is present, and these patients may not be suitable for an office procedure. Consideration for factor replacement with fresh frozen plasma should be given in consultation with a hematologist. Platelet supplementation may also be needed because of thrombocytopenia associated with splenomegaly. The increased INR due to hepatic disease contrasts with the guidelines for treatment of patients on warfarin whereby safe treatment can often be accomplished at levels of 3.5 or less just using local measures. The INR level gives the practitioner a rapid means to assess the degree of hepatic damage.

Renal Disease

As with hepatic disease, the degree of renal failure necessary to trigger clinical signs is significant. Glomerular function can be maintained by adaptive hyperfiltration of the residual nephrons. Once this adaptation is exceeded, signs of renal failure ensue. Clinicians may note fluid overload (pulmonary or peripheral edema), hypertension, anemia, and excessive bruising. Electrolyte disorders, especially hyperkalemia, become problematic, potentially affecting cardiac conduction. Significant hyperkalemia can lead to bradycardia and tall peaked T waves with a loss of the P wave.

The loss of the kidney's ability to reabsorb proteins can lead to a plasma protein deficiency. As noted with hepatic disease, this will increase the potential profundity and duration of action of many anesthetic agents. These findings would lead to a consideration for the use of inhalational agents or rapidly redistributed agents such as propofol. Caution with nonsteroidal anti-inflammatory drugs, codeine, and meperidine is noted because these have water-soluble metabolites and also can cause additional renal damage.[5]

Assessing the degree of renal impairment is based on the patient's creatinine level as well as MET level. As renal disease progresses, the resultant fluid overload and hypertension will cause a reduction in normal activities. In patients with kidney failure on dialysis, consideration for treatment on the day after dialysis is considered to put the patient in their most optimal situation. However, the physiologic toll of renal failure will decrease a patient's resiliency and potentially increase anesthetic complications. Fluid overload can easily occur during an anesthetic, whereas fluid deficits can lead to dramatic hypotension.

Geriatric Patients

With the population of patients living longer through better medical care, the OMS is more likely to treat patients of an older age. It can be reasonably assumed that this population will have a higher instance of medical issues that cumulatively negatively impact the patient's resiliency during an anesthetic (**Box 1**). In general,

---

Box 1
Expected physiologic changes in the geriatric population

General

  ↓ Lean muscle mass

  ↑ Fat stores

  ↓ Blood volume

Central nervous system

  Cerebral atrophy: cognitive impairment, confusion, dementia

  Autonomic impairment: labile blood pressure, impaired thermoregulation, delayed gastric emptying

  Neurotransmitter deficiencies: Parkinson and Alzheimer

Cardiovascular

  Congestive heart failure /coronary artery disease

  Atrial fibrillation

  Hypertension and changes in arterial elasticity (stiffness)

Pulmonary

  Diminished functional reserve: ↓ vital capacity, flattened diaphragms, weak muscles

  Blunted response to ↑ CO_2 or ↓ O_2

  Loss of protective coughing and swallowing reflexes

Renal

  ↓ Growth factor receptor and blood flow to the kidneys

  Fluid and electrolyte imbalance

  ↓ Capacity to excrete drugs and metabolites

Hepatic

  ↓ Blood flow to the liver

  ↓ Ability to metabolize drugs with high E ratio

  ↓ Albumin and protein binding

From Schreiber A, Tan PM. Anesthetic considerations for geriatric patients. In: Bosack R, Lieblich S, editors. Anesthesia complications in dental patients. Ames (IA): Wiley; 2014. p. 98; with permission.

one can anticipate a decline in all the major organ systems as aging occurs. There is no specific age cutoff for an office anesthetic because individuals will substantially vary in the rate of their decline as well as the overall ability of organs to compensate for partial functional loss. Box 1 offers an insight into some of the issues affecting these patients, and of course, more than one system can be involved. Frailty has been described as a predictor of increased surgical risk, which includes a decrease in grip strength, unintentional weight loss (>4.5 kg), exhaustion, and decreased walking speed with reduction in physical activity[6] (again, information that may be gleaned from an evaluation of MET level).

Geriatric patients also have a higher likelihood of being on medications to manage their systemic disease. For example, even with good control of blood pressure with a diuretic, a patient can be more susceptible to hypotension during the induction of an anesthetic or hypervolemia and hypovolemia as well. The practitioner needs to gather a complete list of medications during the initial consultation appointment to determine how stable a patient may be. Valuable information can be also obtained if it is learned that a new medication has recently been started because this indicates a medical condition that may not be fully optimized or that the medication level may not yet be properly titrated.

Many patients will have a list of their medications with them, and verification should be made that no additions or deletions have occurred since they prepared this list. The OMS should verify that indeed the patient is taking their medications as actually prescribed, because, due to financial issues, some patients may not be on their correct schedule of medications. The Beers Criteria is a useful tool for the OMS to evaluate for possible inappropriate medications for the geriatric patient.[7] It is interesting to note that the Beers Criteria also distinguishes the increased risk to a patient taking 5 or more prescriptions. Beer's criteria could be a useful screening tool for the OMS anesthetic patient as well.

As part of the patient's evaluation to undergo an anesthetic, there should also be an evaluation of the preoperative and postoperative care that will be available. Other family members such as a spouse may have even more medical issues and be less able to provide even simple observation postoperatively. Younger family members that attend the consultation appointment should be verified that they will be there for this aspect of care as well.

Pediatric Patients

In contrast to adult patients, the pediatric patient is typically healthier and has less background medical issues. The medical history of a child is obtained from a parent or informed caregiver. If a systemic disorder is present, the child is usually under the care of a physician and it is hoped optimized. However, an abnormal medical condition of a child can have more significant consequences than in an adult because the child has less functional reserve. Similar questions as given to an adult can be asked regarding a child's functional activity, such as participation in sports, activities of daily living, and also the possibility of signs of sleep apnea. Concerns with unrefreshed sleep, reports of snoring, or daytime somnolence can alert the practitioner to the possibility.

Childhood obesity can also be an issue that primarily impacts the OMS in regards to respiration. The long-term consequences of obesity, such as diabetes and coronary artery disease, are not likely to present in a child. Certainly, difficulty in starting an intravenous line for children in general and particularly obese children is an issue.

The preoperative examination of a child needs to include careful auscultation of the lungs because any impairment reduces an already limited capacity. On top of the relatively decreased functional residual capacity, children have narrower airways, which are more prone to collapse.

The preoperative evaluation of a child typically includes the same format as an adult with classification based on ASA status and an airway examination. Other classification schemes have been proposed for children to see if an improved correlation with the need for escalation of care can be predicted. One such pediatric screening tool that has been shown to have a higher correlation for the occurrence of adverse events is the NARCO-SS[8] than even the ASA status. NARCO-SS takes into account the child's neurologic status, airway, respiratory, cardiac, and "other" (endocrine, renal issues, and so forth). The SS refers to surgical severity and for office procedures is assumed to be a low risk of the actual procedure. Although a better correlation exists versus the ASA status, the primary concern in the OMS anesthetic is the airway, and this score does not seem to be as predictable for an adverse outcome.

SUMMARY

The provision of anesthesia in the OMS office is an important part of the overall care provided. This aspect of practice provides the ability of patients to undergo procedures that may have been required to be performed in a hospital or other facility potentially limiting access to care. However, it is incumbent on the OMS to carefully evaluate a patient and to be able to say "no" to an office anesthetic[9] even if the patient demands it. Thorough preoperative patient evaluation is just one aspect of the provision of safe surgical care in the office, but it is the initial part of the process.

REFERENCES

1. Miloro M, Basi D, Halpern L, et al. Patient assessment. In: Sims P, Lieblich SE, editors. Parameters of care: AAOMS clinical guidelines for oral and maxillofacial surgery. 6th edition. J Oral Maxillofac Surg 2017:e12–33.
2. Tait A, Malviya S. Anesthesia for the child with an upper respiratory tract infection: still a dilemma? Anesth Analg 2005;100(1):59–65.
3. Wong J, Lam DP, Abrishami A, et al. Short term preoperative smoking cessation and postoperative complications: a systematic review and meta-analysis. Can J Anaesth 2012;59:268–79.
4. Miller J, Lieblich S. Anesthetic considerations for patients with hepatic disease. In: Bosack R, Lieblich S, editors. Anesthesia complications in dentistry. St Louis (MO): Wiley; 2014. p. 85–9.
5. Levine M, Schreber A. Anesthetic considerations for patients with renal disease. In: Bosack R, Lieblich S, editors. Anesthesia complications in dentistry. St Louis (MO): Wiley; 2014. p. 89–93.
6. Markary MA, Segev DL, Pronovost PJ, et al. Frailty as a predictor of surgical outcomes in older patients. J Am Coll Surg 2010;210(6):901–8.
7. American Geriatric Society updated beers criteria for potentially inappropriate medication use in older adults. Available at: https://geriatricscareonline.org/toc/american-geriatrics-society-updated-beers-criteria-for-potentially-inappropriate-medication-use-in-older-adults/CL001. Accessed July 28, 2017.
8. Udupa AN, Ravindra MN, Chandrika YR, et al. Comparison of pediatric perioperative risk assessment by ASA physical status and by NARCO-SS (neurological, airway, respiratory, cardiovascular, other surgical severity) scores. Paediatr Anaesth 2015;25(3):309–16.
9. Herlich A, Bosack RC. When should you say no?. In: Bosack R, Lieblich S, editors. Anesthesia complications in dentistry. St Louis (MO): Wiley; 2014. p. 315–20.

Oral and Maxillofacial Surgery Team Anesthesia Model and Anesthesia Assistant Training

Stephanie J. Drew, DMD

KEYWORDS

- Oral and maxillofacial surgery office-based team anesthesia • Anesthesia assistant training
- Crisis resource management • AAOMS anesthesia assistant training programs

KEY POINTS

- Safety and efficacy of oral maxillofacial surgery (OMFS) office-based, open airway anesthesia is maximized with a systems-based team approach.
- Anesthesia assistants should receive training to enhance their skill sets.
- The AAOMS currently offers 5 training programs for anesthesia assisting.
- This document should be shared with all members of the anesthesia team.

INTRODUCTION

The practice scope of the anesthesia assistant is ever increasing. The knowledge base encompasses several medical disciplines, as detailed in **Box 1**. As these components are embraced, focus will then turn to the support and participation in the 6 patient safety initiatives, as shown in **Box 2**.

Oral maxillofacial surgery (OMFS) offers various levels of sedation to mitigate anxiety, fear, and discomfort that can be associated with the delivery of care. Nitrous oxide, midazolam, fentanyl, ketamine, and propofol (among others) are currently popular drugs used to achieve these goals. Drug choice and dose are selected to achieve various levels of sedation as shown in **Table 1**. The reader will appreciate that the depth of sedation is a continuum, ranging from the sleepy but otherwise unaffected minimally sedated patient, to the moderately sedated patient who will follow commands and respond appropriately to verbal/tactile stimulation, to the patient under general anesthesia who cannot respond purposefully to any level of stimulation. Further examination of this table will reveal that with deepening levels of sedation, adverse changes involving the ability to maintain an open airway, ability to maintain satisfactory ventilatory rate and depth, and the ability to maintain blood pressure can occur. At any given drug or dose, and in any given patient, movement between these arbitrary levels of sedation can be rapid and unexpected, hence the need for intense and redundant monitoring in order to anticipate impending trouble and permit adequate time for successful remediation. Because of the wide variability of patient response, achieving and maintaining an appropriate level of sedation can be challenging. Because of this, the risk of sedation often becomes greater than the risk of the procedure that it was meant to enable. This risk can be effectively managed by the anesthetic team.

The OMS anesthesia team model is one in which a team is responsible for the care of the patient. The OMS functions as team leader who performs patient selection, the immediate preoperative assessment, and the procedure; additionally, he

Disclosures: None.

Division of Oral and Maxillofacial Surgery, Emory University School of Medicine, 1365 Clifton Road NE, Building B, Suite 2300, Atlanta, GA 30322, USA

E-mail address: Stephanie.drew@emory.edu

oralmaxsurgery.theclinics.com

Box 1
Some components of anesthesia assisting

1. Basics of anatomy, physiology, and pathophysiology, with emphasis on the cardiovascular, pulmonary, and nervous systems
2. Importance of an accurate medical history, as it relates to patient selection and preanesthetic evaluation for office-based sedation
3. Components of safe and effective anesthesia
4. Familiarization with equipment
5. Patient monitoring, during and after sedation
6. Duties for airway maintenance during sedation

---

or she oversees the anesthetic management. The surgical assistant assists with the surgery and has secondary roles in emergency management. The anesthesia assistant's sole duty is to maintain the airway, appraise ventilations, and follow the status of the patient on the patient monitors, especially end tidal CO_2 and secondarily pulse oximetry. A team coordinator is available in emergency management, and this person is responsible for activating emergency medical services (EMS) and frequently serves as a scribe to document actions in emergency management. The OMS anesthesia team model has served the public well and has a good safety record. Optimizing team performance for routine anesthetic care and preparation for emergency management is vital for patient safety.

WHEN THINGS GO WRONG

In an ideal scenario, a patient will present to the OMFS office, tender a written health history, which then is verbally reviewed. A diagnosis and treatment plan will be made; the preanesthetic evaluation will guide the intended level of sedation, and

---

Box 2
Patient safety initiatives for the anesthesia team

1. Culture of safety
2. Conservative patient selection
3. Depth of anesthesia limit setting
4. Intensive, redundant monitoring
5. Basic emergency airway management (discussed in Clive Rayner and Michael R. Ragan's article, "Are You Ready for EMS in Your OMS Office?," in this issue)

---

the patient will be sedated. Then, the procedure will be completed; the patient will recover (wake-up), meet criteria for safe discharge, and return home. In all instances, several staff members become involved with these processes, which require an adequate knowledge base, some level of decision making, and accurate communication.

Sometimes, errors (deviations from safe practice) are made. These mistakes may be caused by individual human error[1,2] (eg, forgetfulness, carelessness, lack of understanding, thought burden, inattention, cover-up) and/or systems (latent) error (eg, poor teamwork, overbooking, lack of team training, lack of protocols, and sloppy information gathering/communication).[1] In most cases, these mistakes will create either an unsafe condition or a near miss; in both instances, harm and injury never reach the patient. However, when a series of errors serendipitously and temporally align, the summation of both mistakes and misfortune can lead to patient injury, otherwise termed a sentinel event, unexpected, unplanned, unintended, and undesirable patient outcomes. This situation is graphically depicted in the now classic Swiss cheese model of accident theory.[3] As shown in **Fig. 1**, the straight line trajectory from a practice deviation (error) to patient injury might have been blocked by the anesthesia team in several ways: communicating compromising patient factors to the OMFS, attentive patient monitoring during anesthesia, and crisis resource management during an emergent situation. Flaws in these safety road blocks are represented by the holes in the Swiss cheese. The importance of the anesthesia team embracing a culture of safety by improving anesthetic safety cannot be overstated.

ANESTHETIC MEDICATION

The type and dose of anesthetic medication are chosen to provide anxiolysis, forgetfulness, pain relief, and sleep, as necessary, to complete the planned oral surgical procedure. As stated previously, drug effect cannot always be accurately predicted, and when drugs are given in combination or repeatedly, the possibility of overdose leading to adverse effects increases. The 3 most important adverse effects all pertain to the inability to deliver oxygen to tissues: loss of upper airway patency, decrease or lack of ventilatory urge, and hypotension (a drop in blood pressure), which then fails to drive blood and oxygen flow to tissues. This is in contradistinction to underdosing, which triggers a fight or flight sympathetic discharge, which can decompensate a compromised heart. The severity and duration of these

Table 1
Continuum of depth of sedation: definition of general anesthesia and levels of sedation/analgesia[a]

	Minimum Sedation (Anxiolysis)	Moderate Sedation/Analgesia (Conscious Sedation)	Deep Sedation/Analgesia	General Anesthesia
Responsiveness	Normal response to verbal stimulation	Purposeful[b] response to verbal or tactile stimulation	Purposeful[b] response after repeated or painful stimulation	Unarousable
Airway	Unaffected	No intervention required	Intervention may be required	Intervention often required
Spontaneous ventilation	Unaffected	Adequate	May be inadequate	Frequently inadequate
Cardiovascular function	Unaffected	Usually maintained	Usually maintained	May be impaired

As sedation is a continuum, individual patient responses are variable and may not exactly follow these categorizations.
Reflex withdrawal from a painful stimulus is not considered a purposeful response.
From American Society of Anesthesiologists Task Force on Sedation and Analgesia by Non-Anesthesiologists. Practice guidelines for sedation and analgesia by non-anesthesiologists. Anaesthesiology 2002;96(4):1005; with permission.

adverse effects affect the patient's ability to tolerate them.

CONSERVATIVE PATIENT SELECTION

Box 3 is a partial list of adverse patient conditions and disease states that can negatively affect their ability to tolerate the stress of anesthesia and surgery. These patients should be carefully scrutinized by the anesthetic team prior to treatment. It remains impossible to scientifically prove that healthier patients are better able to tolerate adverse effects; however, the concept flies with reason. A culture of safety entices all team members to be on the lookout for these compromised patients.

INTENSIVE, REDUNDANT MONITORING

Vigilance is the motto of the American Society of Anesthesiologists.[4] It is defined as the action or state of keeping careful and continuous watch for possible danger or difficulty. Perianesthetic visual patient observation, intermittent blood pressure recording, pulse oximetry, continuous lead II electrocardiography, capnography, and auscultation of the airway give the anesthetic assistant 6 avenues to first anticipate, and then

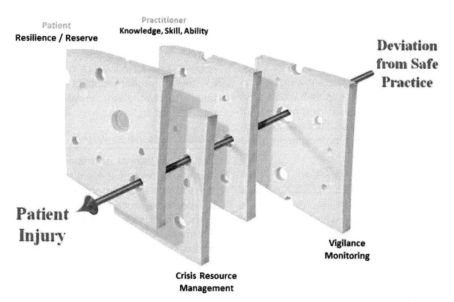

Fig. 1. Swiss cheese model of system accidents.

Box 3
A partial list of patient characteristics that can make them unsuitable for office based anesthesia

1. Upper airway compromise
2. Obstructive sleep apnea
3. Substance abuse disorders
4. Extremes of age
5. Extremes of body weight
6. Active cardiovascular/pulmonary/endocrine disease
7. Poor exercise tolerance

---

rapidly identify any negative change in patient status. This proactive, rather than reactive approach allows early identification, which can minimize the duration and consequence of the insult. Performance decrement is minimized, as time urgency is blunted. A dedicated anesthesia assistant can be easily trained to understand these monitoring modalities and instantly alert the OMFS, who can readily interrupt the procedure and remediate the situation.

CRISIS RESOURCE MANAGEMENT

Crisis resource management is a series of techniques/actions/protocols for managing time-urgent, high-stakes events in the medical environment.[5] These protocols seek to improve the social, team-oriented, nontechnical skills as a viable mechanism to prevent deviations from safe practice from causing patient injury, making the environment (system) more error resistant. By optimizing and utilizing all available resources (eg, self, staff, monitoring, airway devices, cognitive aids, colleagues, paramedics, educational opportunities), the ability to translate knowing what to do into effective performance is enhanced. The following are exemplary salient components of crisis resource management as it applies to sedation safety in the dental office, before, during, and after patient care.[6]

Anticipate and Plan

Consistent with safety culture, practitioners should always plan for the worst. Emergency scenarios should be anticipated, and rescue plans consistent with the nature of the practice should be devised and continually rehearsed by all staff. This is called simulation,[1] which is an enactment of something anticipated, meant to reinforce roles, duties, movement of various

devices, and protocols for management of rare emergency situations. Frequent rehearsal improves retention of these tasks. Errors during simulation do not result in patient harm and can be noted to eliminate their recurrence. During simulation, all team members become aware of their duties and can perform them without waiting for prompts or others to act. The environment can be prepared for the various emergencies. The 3 skill sets that are addressed are affective (interacting), cognitive (thinking), and psychomotor (doing). Affective and cognitive simulation requires participation of the entire team, best accomplished in the office environment (in situ). As each office is unique, individual nuances in diagnosis and treatment protocols can be incorporated. Psychomotor training such as airway interventions, electrical therapy, and auscultation are best practiced on a manikin; however, manikin proficiency does not guarantee human proficiency. The key principle here is practice repeatedly.

Know the Environment

Before commencing any patient treatment, a time out should be taken, where all important features of the case are announced out loud for all to hear, including patient name, health concerns, status, and procedure to be performed. At this time, an equipment check is also done, including monitors, back-up devices, connectors, gas sources, and suction. The plane is on the runway, ready for takeoff.

Use All Available Information

During any emergency, the team leader must perceive and process all pertinent information, including vital signs, status of intravenous access, and patient color. Each team member should know individual responsibilities prior to any emergent situation. Quick glances or fast checks often leave the leader with misinformation.

Allocate Attention Wisely

Optimal situational awareness keeps the practitioner informed of the entire environment, while attending to a single problem. A repeating cycle of perceive-process-perform-perceive-process-perform facilitates movement through a situation. Priorities can be set and changed as needed; reevaluation is frequent, and fixation errors are minimized. During an airway crisis, the first intervention is frequently but sometimes erroneously presumed to be the correct intervention, when it many cases, it is not.

Mobilize Resources

These resources can be additional personnel (colleagues, key staff members), monitors, airway devices, or video laryngoscopes. In any event, at least 1 back-up airway plan should be formulated and immediately available. The rapid identification, location, and movement of equipment to the OMFS is emphasized.

Use Cognitive Aids

Performance decrement during stressful, high-stakes, time-urgent situations occurs almost universally. Mental and sometimes physical *situational paralysis* can occur, grossly interfering with thought processes. During these times, checklists can jog memory and guide direction for crisis resolution. Checklists should be posted in visible locations for all to see. They are most aptly termed simple, shared, structured responses.

Communicate Effectively

During crises, statements or requests are often shouted out, but no one hears. Closed-loop directed communication is most effective (eg, "Mary, please check patient saturation." "Yes, Doctor, I will check saturation, it is ….") Junior team members should not be hesitant to speak up, as authority grids flatten with all intentions focused on patient safety.

Distribute the Workload

The practitioner will need help in urgent times, and will not have the time or inclination to start assigning tasks in the moment of crisis. Staffing should be adequate, informed, and trained, and patient scheduling should be unhurried. All staff should be cross-trained and ready to act without prompting from others.

Call for Help Early

There is no shame in calling for help, such as colleagues or activation of the EMS. It is always better to be safe than sorry, and this action should be praised. It does not indicate a lack of qualification. Interaction with EMS is discussed in Clive Rayner and Michael R. Ragan's article, "Are You Ready for EMS in Your OMS Office?," in this issue.

RESOURCES AVAILABLE FOR ASSISTANT TRAINING

There are a variety of resources available for anesthesia assistant training, and these are listed in **Box 4**. The Office Anesthesia Evaluation Manual is a reference for the OMS anesthesia team and

---

Box 4
Resources available for assistant training

Office anesthesia evaluation manual

Anesthesia assistants review course

Advance protocols for medical emergency

Anesthesia assistants' skills lab

AAOMS simulation program

---

reviews preoperative evaluation, disease processes, emergency management, and facility and equipment standards.

The AAOMS anesthesia assistants review course (AARC) was designed to start at the beginning, basic training. This intensive review course focuses on principles of anesthesia learned through structured training, as well as the latest innovations and methods of anesthesia administration, monitoring, and emergency management. Participants expand their knowledge of basic sciences, patient evaluation and preparation, anesthetic drugs and techniques, and emergency procedures to achieve better patient care. The AARC was developed by the American Association of Oral and Maxillofacial Surgeons; this course is taught by AAOMS fellows and members. It is typically given twice per year. It can also be done online.

The goals of the course are to describe the concepts of medical evaluation of patients for anesthesia, discuss the mechanical and pharmacologic aspects of outpatient anesthesia, and explain the methods of patient monitoring and management of medical emergencies.

This comprehensive review course includes several topics, which will be discussed in the following sections.

Basic Sciences

The class provides information on basic anatomy and physiology. This may be the first time a surgical assistant is exposed to this information. Anatomy and physiology of cardiovascular, pulmonary, circulatory, and central and peripheral nervous systems are presented. Each body system is reviewed in relationship to what one does on a daily basis in the oral surgery practice. The cardiac, respiratory, nervous, endocrine, renal, hepatic, and immune systems are each reviewed relative to anesthetic techniques and the potential emergencies that may arise relative to the system discussed. The information is then made relevant to real issues that may be seen through case examples.

The anatomy of the airway, the heart, and the vascular system, especially as it pertains to intravenous access is a key learning point in this series. Intravenous access is the most utilized path to delivering anesthetic drugs, as well as rescue medications to resuscitate a patient if necessary. The assistants are taught that the intravenous line should be maintained throughout the sedation and until the patient is no longer at risk for cardiorespiratory depression.

Patient Evaluation and Preparation

The ASA recommends that the clinician/team should be familiar with the impact of the patient's medical history and how it may alter the patient's response to sedation/analgesia delivered in the office. The course places emphasis on patients with such medical problems as cardiac, pulmonary, and metabolic diseases. The impact of each disease within the system discussed is presented in a way that highlights the effect on surgery and anesthetic technique and management, as well as the potential emergencies that may arise during or after surgery because of the patient's presenting health conditions.

Key issues that can impact anesthetic technique are abnormalities of a major organ system, previous adverse experiences with sedation, drug allergies, current medications and potential drug interactions, time and the nature of the patient's last oral intake, and history of tobacco, alcohol or substance use. As an anesthetic team member, the basic evaluation skills of recording vital signs must be mastered including taking blood pressure, listening to the lungs, and performing both a preoperative, perioperative, and postoperative airway assessment (see **Fig. 1**).

Anesthetic Drugs and Techniques

Up-to-date information on drugs used in administration of local anesthetic, intravenous sedation, and general anesthesia are presented in the AARC. The course provides the staff with baseline knowledge of the pharmacology of the drugs used each day. The anesthesia assistant team member should be able to identify the drug and be able to note the dose needed with proper labeling on the medication containers and proper route of administration, know how to open the ampules or draw up the medication, and know how to dilute it if needed. The impact that each drug has on the systems is discussed and the potential adverse effects of their use.

The anesthesia assistant must learn that the primary cause of morbidity associated with sedation/analgesia is drug-induced respiratory depression and airway obstruction. The combined use of opioids and sedatives produces effective moderate sedation in this patient population. Each drug given should be administered individually to achieve the desired effect. Sufficient time should be allowed to lapse between dosing to allow the effect to be assessed before additional dosing. This way techniques can be titrated to a safe level of consciousness and sedation.

For the team to be safe and effective, the goal is to set up the anesthesia drugs used to sedate a patient in a systematic way so that there are no errors in delivery. Creating labeled syringes with proper concentration is an important safety step. Ready references (cognitive aids) should be available for the staff, listing drug characteristics (eg, the timing between doses needed if applicable, the maximum dose allowed per patient, the type of syringe needed to draw up the drug, such as "Midazolam (sedative(anxiolytic)) 1 mg/cc. Use 5 cc syringe. Max dose 5 mg. Onset about 2 minutes").

In addition to the sedation medications, the crash cart medications should be set up the same way. The components of a crash cart are presented during the AARC. Methods of organizing the cart are presented so that it is set up in a way so that drugs are organized by emergency. For example, if an allergic reaction occurs, the team can open the cart and go to the section that may house the allergic reaction medications such as diphenhydramine, steroids, and epinephrine. Each drug is labeled with its indications for use in an emergency.

Monitoring

The basic knowledge about the machines we use to monitor patients is presented during the AARC so staff can learn how each piece of equipment is used properly and how to maintain equipment. The basic equipment needed to monitor and maintain safe practices during sedation includes a precordial stethoscope, a pulse oximeter, the capnograph monitor, blood pressure machine or manual sphygmomanometer, and the electrocardiograph. The assistant team member should be able to place these monitors on correctly, and be able to alert the doctor of any dangerous trends. The course instruction will allow the assistant to recognize a normal electrocardiogram from an abnormal one.

If the need to defibrillate arises, most offices today are using an automatic external defibrillator. However, the ability to cardiovert a patient is lacking, and full advanced cardiovascular life support (ACLS) protocol is not possible with an automated external defibrillator (AED). Knowledge in the use of a defibrillator, the energy levels, and set up are important if the need to use energy for an arrest situation is indicated.

Emergency Procedures

The goal of the AARC course is to recognize an anesthesia emergency and discuss what could have been done to prevent it. Presentations of various emergency situations and appropriate treatment plans are presented. The information is then presented using various scenarios that may occur in the office in an emergent situation. Diagnosis of the emergency, treatment with team roles and care guides, emergency record, and safety-based communication methods are presented.

The roles in these emergent situations will be the team leader (usually the doctor), the first assistant in managing the patient directly, the second assistant who will retrieve any needed equipment or drugs and be able to assist in cardiopulmonary resuscitation (CPR), the documenter/communicator to the EMS system. This person should be able to document in real time what is happening and speak with the EMS personnel. How to alert of the emergency medical system (EMS) should be part of the preparedness drills in the office setting. Emergency records should be made up that can be easily accessed to chart the event details including name of the patient, age (date of birth), allergies, drugs that have been delivered, and what has transpired. The address of the office, the phone number, and a second phone number such as a cell phone in case the office loses power.

Airway adjuncts such as bag valve mask techniques are introduced during the AARC along with the use of connectors to deliver medications, nasopharyngeal airways, oral airways and supraglottic airways and endotracheal tubes. The task of managing the setup of an oxygen tank is essential for all team members. Understanding how and when to use these different airway tools by the assistant and doctor will help the team in an emergent situation. Team members will know what to deliver to the doctor when asked for the piece of equipment and also know how to place it themselves if the doctor is otherwise occupied with a different emergent task. This is an important concept with the AAOMS team model.

The next educational offering for assistants is to introduce the specific details of the emergencies that may occur in the office and develop a systematic way to react then treat them as a team. This course is called the AAOMS Advanced Protocols for Medical Emergency (APME) course. The

AAOMS has stated the goal of this program is for the participants to learn how to be able to

1. Recognize potential and real emergencies
2. Evaluate the underlying cause(s) of emergency situations
3. Plan appropriate responses to specific emergencies
4. Function as an integral part of the oral and maxillofacial surgery team to manage office emergencies

This emergency preparedness course also begins with a review of airway emergencies, then review of the cardiac, neurologic, then immune/allergy, then endocrine and hematologic systems. The course ends with the emergency preparedness program and preparation and maintenance of the crash carts. The OODA loop certainly plays a role in this course. Again, scenarios are presented such that practice can be achieved and application of these materials in a group format. Decision trees are discussed and practices for each emergency scenario. It is an exciting course as the surgical assistant now gets to further apply his or her increasing knowledge base related to sedation and emergencies and understanding the prevention of them, further validating the goal of creating a culture of safety.

As part of the emergency protocols, the discussion of reversal agents as part of the crash cart are presented. The team must remember only the opioids and benzodiazepines are reversible. Naloxone is used to reverse opioid-induced sedation and respiratory depression. The anesthesia assistant team member must know the limitations of this medication. Special attention to use of this drug in relation to the reversal of the respiratory depressant effects but may also result in pain, hypertension, tachycardia, or pulmonary edema. Flumazenil is used to reverse the effects of the benzodiazepine-induced sedation and ventilatory depression. The medications may wear off, and the patient may become resedated, causing respiratory depression to present again.

It is recommended that the assistant have taken the AARC course as a primer for the APME. The course can also be taken after the Dental Anesthesia Assistant National Certification Examination (DAANCE) self-study is done; however it is in the author's opinion that the details learned from the AAPME class will help also prepare for the DAANCE examination.

The final phase of anesthesia assistant preparedness training is the simulation of emergencies for the staff to practice on the mannequins in the AAOMS anesthesia assistants' skills laboratory. Participants rotate through 6 stations to include airway management, intubation, venipuncture (including the use of an intraosseous access portal), defibrillation, preparation of emergency drugs, and minicode. Furthermore, registrants are exposed to various airway adjuncts, critical cardiac dysrhythmias and defibrillation, and the use of the peak flow meter and glucometer. Here the laboratory is set up into respiratory and cardiac stations. Teams of anesthesia assisting staff practice different emergency scenarios. The teams are exposed to emergencies that may lead to cardiac events, or respiratory events such as airway obstruction, as well as situations including syncope and insulin overdose, adrenal crisis, and anaphylaxis.

The AAOMS objectives of the skills laboratories are as follows

Recognize airway obstruction, describe its management, and utilize the principal airway adjuncts
Recognize critical cardiac dysrhythmias and demonstrate appropriate management with medications and defibrillation technique; they are taught how to use the AED
Explain the importance of team management of office emergencies; job descriptions for each team member are reviewed at this time
Demonstrate the preparation and administration of emergency drugs and use of diagnostic devices such as the peak flow meter and glucometer; dilution of drugs and the use of the intraosseous bone access for the delivery of medications and fluids is presented

Through a team approach, the assistants each get to function as a team leader are asked to diagnose the problem through their assessment and run through the decision trees as a team leader. They each get a turn in this capacity, and the others are assisting with CPR, drawing up drugs, or documenting the event. They are exposed to various changes in vital signs as well as electrocardiograph monitor changes. They learn how to manage the airway from head position to a cricothyroidotomy. They learn how to help with a "shockable rhythm". While this is a controlled environment for learning, the practice is invaluable to the assistants. They will gain the confidence through education and practice to help you manage the patients through these emergencies.

The ultimate competency assessment of these new anesthesia assisting surgical skills and knowledge is through the (DAANCE). To prepare for this examination, after taking the previous courses, a self-study book is delivered to the candidate and his or her sponsoring surgeon. It takes about 36 hours of reading to go through each of these modules. It is recommended to set aside at least 30 minutes each time one goes through the materials with an assistant. This can be done at breakfast meeting or the end of the day or even lunch type of learning session. The sponsoring doctor must commit to this time for the staff to truly learn the materials. The modules covered are

Basic sciences
Evaluation and preparation of patient with systemic diseases
Anesthetic drugs and techniques
Anesthesia equipment and monitoring
Office anesthesia emergencies

Several practice examinations are also provided as a resource to prepare for the examination. The answers to the practice examinations are given to the sponsoring surgeon. The actual examination is a 2-hour computer-based multiple choice examination given once the self-study is completed. There is a 6-month time limit to take this examination once the candidate registers to take the examination. Passing of this examination then provides the candidate with a certificate of completion and certification.

Ultimately the final team training and preparation will be with the individual team to practice in a real emergency simulation laboratory; then one can bring the skills back to the office. The new AAOMS Office Anesthesia Simulation Course was developed for this purpose and is reviewed in David W. Todd, and John J. Schaefer III article, "The American Association of Oral and Maxillofacial Surgeons (AAOMS) Simulation Program" in this issue. This 3-part program was developed to test office teams in a standardized way in each emergency situation, then assess the areas of strength and deficiency so that the team can improve its performance. Competency comes with deliberate practice.

In conclusion, the OMS team anesthesia model is one in which the OMS functions as team leader and has trained assistants with defined roles, helping to manage the patient in a safe and predictable manner during anesthetic delivery. Conservative patient selection, understanding the levels of sedation, and proper medication management aid a culture of safety in office-based anesthesia delivery. The trained anesthesia assistant has a role solely dedicated to maintaining the airway and monitoring oxygenation and ventilation. In an emergency, team members must utilize their training and practice principles of crew resource management to produce a successful management outcome. There are a variety of training resources and training courses available for anesthesia assistants to increase proficiency in anesthesia delivery and emergency management.

REFERENCES

1. Ostergaard D, Dieckmann P, Lippert A. Simulation and CRM. Best Pract Res Clin Anaesthesiol 2011; 25(2):239–49.
2. Cooper JB, Newbower RS, Kitz RJ. An analysis of major errors and equipment failures in anesthesia management: considerations for prevention and detection. Anesthesiology 1984;60:34–42.
3. Reason J. Human error: models and management. Br Med J 2000;320(3):768–70.
4. Bacon DR. Iconography in anesthesiology. The importance of society seals in the 1920s and 30s. Anesthesiology 1996;85:414–9.
5. Howard SK, Gaba DM, Fish KJ, et al. Anesthesia crisis resource training: teaching anesthesiologists to handle critical incidents. Aviat Space Environ Med 1992;63:763–70.
6. Rall M, Dieckmann P. Safety culture and crisis resource management in airway management: general principles to enhance patient safety in critical airway situations. Best Pract Res Clin Anaesthesiol 2005;19(4):539–57.

Anesthetic Agents Commonly Used by Oral and Maxillofacial Surgeons

Kyle J. Kramer, DDS, MS[a],*, Jason W. Brady, DMD[b,c,1]

KEYWORDS

- Midazolam • Diazepam • Ketamine • Dexmedetomidine • Propofol • Nitrous oxide
- Anesthetic agents • Inhalational

KEY POINTS

- Thorough knowledge and understanding of an anesthetic agent's pharmacodynamic and pharmacokinetic profile are critical for safe and efficient clinical use.
- Short-acting drugs without active metabolites are ideal for providing the full spectrum of anesthesia in the unique office-based dental environment.
- To maximize satisfactory outcomes, selected anesthetic agents must match well with the needs of the patient, anticipated procedure, and surgeon.

INTRODUCTION

The oral and maxillofacial surgeon providing full-spectrum dental anesthesia services in the office-based environment currently has a multitude of anesthetic options available. In fact, this may be the dawn of a new "golden age of anesthesia" because of the novel agents and techniques being discovered that can quickly render a patient unconscious yet also provide an extremely fast and smooth emergence and recovery profile ideal for the unique dental environment. The multitude of options available today provide practitioners with great flexibility to create an individualized anesthetic plan, balancing the risks inherent with the patient's medical history and the anticipated surgical plan to achieve maximal results.

BENZODIAZEPINES: DIAZEPAM, MIDAZOLAM, REMIMAZOLAM

Since the discovery of chlordiazepoxide in 1957, benzodiazepines have had a strong presence in dental anesthesia, because of their relatively wide therapeutic index and low risk of producing unconsciousness and respiratory depression when administered alone at modest doses. It took time for the addictive profile of benzodiazepines to become apparent, after which rampant, unmonitored use was brought under further control and scrutiny. Nevertheless, benzodiazepines remain popular sedative and anxiolytic agents. There are currently dozens of available benzodiazepines that may be used for a multitude of purposes; however, a select few are more commonly used for anesthesia (**Table 1**).

Disclosure Statement: The authors have nothing to disclose at this time.
a Department of Oral Surgery and Hospital Dentistry, Indiana University School of Dentistry, 550 North University Boulevard, Room UH3143, Indianapolis, IN 46202, USA; b Department of Dental Anesthesia, NYU Langone Hospital, 150 55th Street, Brooklyn, NY 11220, USA; c Division of Endodontics, Orthodontics and General Practice Residency, Herman Ostrow School of Dentistry of USC, 925 West 34th Street, Los Angeles, CA 90089, USA
1 Present address: 3343 East Indigo Bay, Gilbert, AZ 85234.
* Corresponding author.
E-mail address: kjkramer@iu.edu

Table 1 Benzodiazepines	
Initial IV dosing[a]	
Diazepam	2.5–5 mg
Midazolam	1–2 mg
Oral dosing	
Diazepam	2–10 mg orally
Midazolam	0.5 mg/kg; 20 mg maximum

[a] Titrated to desired effect.

Pharmacodynamics

Benzodiazepines all act as gamma-aminobutyric acid (GABA) -positive allosteric modulators, facilitating the ease at which GABA can bind to its own respective twin binding sites on neuronal chloride ion channels. What makes benzodiazepines unique is not the net increase in GABA activity or inhibitory neuronal activity, but rather the fact that they have their own binding site, called the benzodiazepine receptor, which is found on the gamma subunit of the chloride ion channel. When benzodiazepines bind to this benzodiazepine binding site, it causes a conformational shift in the spatial alignment of the subunits making up the chloride ion channel. The net result is an uncovering of one of the $GABA_A$ receptors, which permits GABA neurotransmitters easier access to their binding sites. Once both $GABA_A$ receptors are engaged and activated by GABA, the previously closed chloride ion channel opens, permitting the influx of chloride ions into the neuron, negatively hyperpolarizing the cell. Interestingly, to date there are no other known agonists for the benzodiazepine binding site; however, several other anesthetic agents do function in a similar fashion producing $GABA_A$-positive allosteric modulation albeit via alternative binding sites. In addition, benzodiazepines have the added benefit of a competitive antagonist, flumazenil, which is capable of reversing the activity of benzodiazepines.

All benzodiazepines produce dose-dependent central nervous system (CNS) depression ranging from anxiolysis to general anesthesia. Benzodiazepines are capable of producing anterograde amnesia, although this effect can be variable and should not be guaranteed. Despite the fact that benzodiazepines cause global CNS depression, they have also been known to cause paradoxic excitatory reactions in some patients, with the highest risk associated with extremes of age. From a cardiovascular and respiratory standpoint, benzodiazepines tend to be rather safe when used alone in modest doses. A minimal reduction in systemic vascular resistance may be appreciated, which is mainly attributed to the anxiolytic effects and decreased

sympathetic outflow. Benzodiazepines cause minimal depression of the respiratory drive, especially when given as a solo agent. However, this safe profile is ablated when used concurrently with other CNS depressant drugs producing synergistic or additive effects. Benzodiazepines also produce centrally mediated skeletal muscle relaxation, which can contribute to collapse of the airway musculature, upper airway obstruction, and loss of airway patency.

Pharmacokinetics

The pharmacokinetics of benzodiazepines depends not only on the specific agent but also the route of administration, with the onset speed being the fastest in parenteral routes, followed by the considerably slower enteral routes. Benzodiazepines are metabolized hepatically, typically via a variety of agent-specific cytochrome p450 enzymes, most commonly the 3A4 or 2D6 isozyme variety.[1]

Diazepam notoriously has several active byproducts, all of which can significantly extend the duration of action such that a "hangover" effect may persist for days. The longest is desmethyldiazepam, which has an elimination half-life approximating 36 to 200 hours.[1] Oxazepam and temazepam, 2 of its other active metabolites, are benzodiazepines as well and can persist for considerable lengths of time. Midazolam has an active metabolite, α-hydroxymidazolam; however, its short half-life makes it clinically insignificant. Diazepam and midazolam can be administered enterally or parenterally. As enteral agents, they are subject to first pass hepatic metabolism as well as the modulation effects concurrently found with CYP450 isozyme inhibitors or inducers. Remimazolam is an ultra-short-acting benzodiazepine currently in phase 3 clinical trials, but is likely to play a significant role in office-based anesthesia in the near future. It is metabolized via tissue esterases, rather than undergoing hepatic metabolism, and has the added benefits of lacking active metabolites or accumulating in the peripheral tissues. Its pharmacokinetic profile essentially mimics that of remifentanil, only exerting activity for ~5 to 10 minutes before all effects begin to wane completely. Theoretically, such a drug could be used to thoroughly sedate a patient, only to have them recover completely in an extremely short period of time. Remimazolam is worthy of attention with regards to future trends in ambulatory anesthesia.

Clinical Use

Diazepam can be given orally to reduce preoperative anxiety either the night before or an hour before the patient's appointment. Avoidance of any other CNS depressant medications is recommended for patients in unmonitored settings. Oral midazolam has been used primarily for pediatric patients to facilitate not only preoperative anxiolysis but also procedural sedation. One potential drawback of the routine use of preoperative oral benzodiazepines is the prolonged onset time. Although there is a high degree of variability, the onset time approximates 45 to 60 minutes, with the peak effect time being highly variable as well. This delayed onset of enterally administered drugs severely hampers accurate titration. Clinicians may select alternate routes of administration to improve efficiency, reserving enteral benzodiazepines for those patients with such significant preoperative anxiety that they may not be otherwise capable of arriving to the office.

Diazepam and midazolam both can be readily titrated to a desired clinical level of sedation/anesthesia via the intravenous (IV) route. The onset for IV diazepam and midazolam tends to be relatively quick with sedative effects being noted within 1.5 to 2 minutes. However, the peak effect tends to be more delayed, approximating 3 to 5 minutes. As such, clinicians should titrate slowly to avoid accidental overdose. Diazepam is not water soluble; hence, the solvent propylene glycol is required to render it suitable for IV/intramuscular (IM) administration. It can be irritating to patients, who may complain of burning, and has been associated with multiple reports of venous thrombosis. Midazolam does not contain this additive and thus does not carry the same complication risk. There is a subtle, yet appreciable difference in the clinical profile produced by either agent. Diazepam tends to produce profound anxiolysis and significant skeletal muscle relaxation; patients often demonstrate the Verrill sign, indicating they remain awake but are extremely relaxed. Midazolam also is potent anxiolytic, but patients more often demonstrate a stronger sedative profile, resting quietly, typically with eyes closed. Similar differences may be appreciated among other benzodiazepines because their clinical profiles are all somewhat individualized and distinct. Benzodiazepines are very effective agents for halting seizure activity.

PROPOFOL

Since its clinical introduction in 1977, propofol (2,6-diisopropylphenol) has become a mainstay for IV induction and maintenance.[2] Propofol is a sedative/hypnotic capable of producing amnesia but notoriously lacking any analgesic properties. It has a very rapid onset, short duration of action, and clean emergence profile that has made it an especially popular anesthetic agent, particularly for sedation and anesthesia in the ambulatory office-based environment (**Table 2**).

Table 2 Propofol	
Induction of general anesthesia	
IV bolus	1.5–2.5 mg/kg
Maintenance of sedation/general anesthesia	
Continuous infusion	100–200 µg/kg/min (deep sedation/general anesthesia) 25–50 µg/kg/min (moderate sedation)
Antiemetic/PONV prophylaxis	
Continuous infusion	15–20 µg/kg/min
Bolus	0.5–1 mg/kg; given 15 min before end of case
Rescue for active PONV	
Bolus	10–20 mg; titrate slowly to effect

Pharmacodynamics

Propofol is a positive allosteric modulator of GABA, involving $GABA_A$ receptors on chloride ion channels. The net result is the same as with barbiturates and benzodiazepines; however, propofol has its own specific binding site unrelated to the aforementioned anesthetic agents. Propofol's extremely rapid onset produces smooth inductions within 30 to 60 seconds of IV administration, due to its high degree of lipophilicity. Propofol has a narrow therapeutic index capable of causing dose-dependent global CNS depression ranging from anxiolysis to general anesthesia. It is notable not only for its antiemetic properties but also for its association with seizurelike phenomenon, which is most commonly appreciated during induction or emergence.[3] In addition to its sedative/hypnotic effects, propofol causes dose- and rate-dependent respiratory and cardiovascular depression, manifesting as hypotension, bradycardia, reduced respiratory rate, tidal volume, and airway muscle tone.[4] Similar to most other anesthetic agents, concurrent use with other CNS depressants is known to cause significant synergistic or additive effects.

Pharmacokinetics

Propofol has a short duration of clinical activity due to its large volume of distribution and lipophilicity, with a redistribution half-life of 2 to 8 minutes.[5] Propofol is hepatically metabolized using glucuronidation and sulfate conjugation mechanisms.[6] The degree of elimination tends to exceed hepatic blood flow, which suggests it likely has extrahepatic metabolic pathways, which have not been completely identified as of yet.[7] The elimination half-life of propofol is a 3 to 12 hours, but it lacks any appreciable active metabolites, which facilitates a smooth recovery free from any lingering effects.[8–10] The pharmacokinetic profile of propofol is such that it can easily be titrated to the desired effect without any appreciable concern for prolonged clinical activity.

Clinical Use

Propofol is extremely popular for IV inductions and as a maintenance agent for total intravenous anesthesia (TIVA) techniques. Propofol is commonly mixed with other anesthetic agents, such as remifentanil or ketamine in one syringe. Although there is one study suggesting the immiscibility of propofol necessitating the use of separate syringes and pumps to maintain consistency of drug delivery,[11] clinical significance of immiscibility has not been established when drug mixtures are being infused over short periods of time. Propofol's antiemetic properties make it an excellent alternative to traditional inhalational anesthetics. It can be used to help reduce the risk of postoperative nausea and vomiting (PONV), especially when used in combination with other PONV-reducing strategies, such as opioid avoidance. The antiemetic benefits of propofol typically last only a few hours after discontinuation of the drug; therefore, propofol is most ideal when used for initial prevention. However, patients who are nauseous or actively vomiting but unresponsive to other PONV modalities (5-HT$_3$ receptor antagonists, phenothiazines) may respond well to small boluses of propofol.

KETAMINE

Ketamine is a dissociative anesthetic that causes dose-dependent sedation and anesthesia via uncoupling of the limbic and thalamoneocortical systems.[10] This rather unique pharmacodynamic action produces a clinical profile that is markedly different compared with most other anesthetic agents. After administration, patients often display a unique cataleptic state or stare, with significantly diminished responsiveness and purposeful movement. Respiratory drive and airway reflexes usually are unaffected and remain intact. Additional findings can include nystagmus and increased salivation. Ketamine has a high degree of bioavailability, which permits its use via enteral and parenteral routes, although IV and IM routes are clinically preferred. It is an ideal agent for IM inductions for patients who are otherwise unable to tolerate placement of a peripheral venous catheter, such as pre-cooperative pediatric or special needs patients.

Pharmacodynamics/Pharmacokinetics

Ketamine is a phencyclidine derivative that acts primarily as a noncompetitive glutamate receptor antagonist, more specifically involving the receptor subtype N-methyl-D-aspartate (NMDA) (**Table 3**). However, it has several additional pharmacodynamic sites of action that are reviewed in later discussion. Although some reports of ketamine precipitating epileptiform or seizure activity have been published, it is generally considered safe for patients with a positive seizure history, especially if combined with other CNS depressants.[12] Ketamine causes very few pulmonary effects when given alone; however, if administered with other CNS depressants, it can potentiate depression of the respiratory drive. It is also capable of causing bronchial smooth muscle relaxation, which is primarily due to inhibition of vagal nerve activity more so than beta-adrenergic action, via inhibition of catecholamine reuptake.[13] Ketamine causes direct negative myocardial inotropic effects; however, this is balanced out by dose-dependent direct CNS stimulation that produces a net increase in sympathetic outflow. The end result is that ketamine clinically produces mild to modest increases in systemic and pulmonary vascular resistance, heart rate, and overall myocardial workload.

Ketamine is relatively lipophilic and has a fairly quick onset approximating 30 to 60 seconds with a peak effect in 1 to 5 minutes for the IV route and an onset of 2 to 3 minutes with a peak effect between 5 and 15 minutes for the IM route.[14–16] The duration of the clinical effects following the initial administration of ketamine depends primarily on the route and the dose. However, ketamine has a relatively brief redistribution half-life of 11

Table 3 Ketamine sites of action	
Site of Action	**Activity**
NMDA	Noncompetitive antagonist
Nicotinic acetylcholine	Negative allosteric modulator
Opioid (μ, κ, δ subtypes)	Weak/very weak agonist
Dopamine (D2)	Agonist
Muscarinic acetylcholine	Antagonist
Serotonin, dopamine, norepinephrine	Reuptake inhibitor
Voltage-gated Na$^+$ channel	Channel blockade
L-type Ca^{++} channel	Channel blockade

to 16 minutes and a terminal half-life of 2 to 3 hours, both of which may be attributed to its very large volume of distribution as well as its rapid hepatic clearance, biotransformation, and renal excretion.[17,18] As mentioned previously, ketamine is metabolized by the liver primarily via N-demethylation by cytochrome p450 enzymes, of which CYP3A4 is the main contributor.[19] The breakdown of ketamine produces several metabolites, the most important being the active byproduct norketamine, which is ~33% as potent as ketamine and ultimately converted into the inactive metabolite dehydronorketamine.[20,21] When administered via parenteral routes, ketamine undergoes significant first-pass hepatic metabolism.

Clinical Use

Ketamine is quite effective for the induction and maintenance of anesthesia through a variety of means, although the most common are IV or IM administration (**Table 4**). Special dosing considerations must be given because the risk of postanesthetic complications is directly related to the total dose of ketamine administered. Significant side effects, such as postoperative nausea and vomiting, emergence delirium, hallucinations, hypersalivation, or prolonged nystagmus, are more common with IM doses greater than 4 mg/kg.[22,23] Similar complications can be appreciated following large single boluses or extended continuous infusions of ketamine. As with all anesthetic drugs, use of the smallest effective dose is recommended to avoid these complications. IV administration of subanesthetic doses of ketamine can be quite useful as anesthetic adjuncts for patients with higher anesthetic requirements. Patients on chronic opioid medications (eg, chronic pain patients) often benefit from the addition of a small subanesthetic bolus of ketamine. The analgesic effects of the added ketamine are often quite beneficial in maintaining a "smooth" anesthetic course. In addition, the use of small boluses of ketamine can help avoid the increased risk of the aforementioned postanesthetic side effects or complications. Finally, the use of ketamine as a preemptive analgesic remains controversial within the dental/oral surgical literature. Investigators have both supported and denied that use of ketamine before the surgical insult helps reduce pain within the first 24 hours for patients following oral surgical procedures.[24,25]

ALPHA-2 AGONISTS (DEXMEDETOMIDINE)

Alpha-2 adrenergic agonists, particularly dexmedetomidine, have anxiolytic, sedative/hypnotic, analgesic, and sympatholytic properties that can be used to manage hypertension, attention-deficit disorder, anxiety, migraines, and withdrawal from alcohol and opioids.[26] The use of alpha-2 agonists for perioperative sedation is increasing in popularity because of their ability to reduce anesthetic requirements and minimize pretreatment anxiety and emergence delirium, while maintaining respiratory drive and airway reflexes.

Pharmacodynamics

Alpha-2 agonists activate secondary and tertiary protein messenger systems that ultimately cause the inhibition of adenylyl cyclase, causing the decreased production of intracellular cyclic adenosine monophosphate, which modulates the synaptic vesicle release of neurotransmitters, primarily norepinephrine (**Fig. 1**). They act centrally to produce hypnotic effects at the locus ceruleus of the brain stem and analgesic effects within the spinal cord.[27] Hemodynamic alterations stem from activation of the central acting α_2 adrenoceptors within the vasomotor centers of the medulla, reducing sympathetic outflow and inhibiting cardiac output by decreasing chronotropic, inotropic, and dromotropic effects on the heart as well as causing vasoconstriction and vasodilation. It

Table 4		
Ketamine		
Induction/procedural sedation		
IV bolus	0.5–1.5 mg/kg
IM bolus	3 mg/kg (2–5 mg/kg)
Acute analgesic adjunct		
IV subanesthetic bolus	0.25 mg/kg

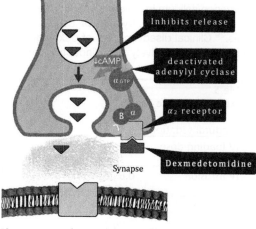

Fig. 1. Dexmedetomidine: mechanism of action. cAMP, cyclic adenosine monophosphate; GTP, guanosine triphosphate.

elicits a biphasic response causing short-lived hypertension and then hypotension. Dexmedetomidine is one of the most highly selective α_2 agonists available, with an affinity ratio of 1620:1 for $\alpha_2{:}\alpha_1$, and although it shares physiologic similarities with clonidine, its affinity for α_2 is 7 times higher than clonidine.[28] The predictable and stable hemodynamic effects without respiratory depression provide optimal benefits for anesthesia providers. It also acts as an antisialagogue, has opioid-sparing effects, and is neuroprotective, but is not as potent of an amnesic agent as benzodiazepines.

Pharmacokinetics

IV dexmedetomidine has a fairly rapid onset within 5 minutes and peak effect within 15 minutes. Dexmedetomidine is rapidly distributed, with a short redistribution half-life of 6 minutes, and undergoes hepatic metabolism, producing inactive metabolites mainly via glucuronidation and hydroxylation, with an elimination half-life of ~2 hours. Despite being designed for IV use only, it is well absorbed through the nasal and buccal mucosa. Intranasal delivery lacks any burning sensation so pediatric patients may tolerate intranasal dexmedetomidine to a higher degree than intranasal midazolam.[29,30]

Clinical Use

Dexmedetomidine has a variety of clinical uses, including preoperative sedation, attenuation of hemodynamic responses to intraoperative stresses, intensive care unit sedation, controlled hypotension, and for procedural sedation. When used as the sole agent via continuous infusion, the loading dose is administered over 10 minutes, which facilitates a speedier onset, although avoidance can minimize hemodynamic alterations (**Table 5**). It can also be used to decrease the incidence of emergence delirium in children without prolonging the time to discharge by use of subanesthetic doses.[29] Clinical disadvantages of dexmedetomidine include a relatively slow induction time to

avoid hemodynamic changes, and a variable quality of sedation among patients. The sedative profile produced by dexmedetomidine is similar to that associated with sleep. Constant surgical stimulation, common in many oral surgical procedures, can lead to spontaneous arousal. Cost remains a primary disincentive; however, the US Food and Drug Administration has recently approved a generic version of Precedex.

OPIOID AGONISTS: MORPHINE, HYDROMORPHONE, FENTANYL CONGENERS

Perioperative administration of opioids has long been used to provide analgesia, typically in combination with other sedative/hypnotic agents facilitating a multimodal or balanced anesthetic approach. Opioids inhibit the upward flow of noxious stimuli from the periphery, thereby reducing the "pain signal" ultimately received by the brain. In addition, opioids are quite effective at offsetting the reduction in the pain threshold noted with several other sedative/hypnotic agents. There are a multitude of opioids (endogenous, opium alkaloids, semisynthetic, synthetic); however, morphine, hydromorphone, and the fentanyl congeners are most common, with profiles that mesh well with the needs accompanying oral surgical procedures.

Pharmacodynamics

Opioids produce analgesia by activating opioid receptors within the dorsal horn of the spinal cord, the medulla, and cortex, and to a lesser degree, peripheral sensory nerves. This activation inhibits afferent noxious neuronal transmission, potentiates the modulation of descending inhibitory pain pathways, and decreases the perception and emotional response to pain.[31] Several opioid receptors have been identified with the $\mu/\delta/\kappa$ subtypes being the prototypical examples capable of producing their own clinical effects. The $\mu2$ subtype is particularly notable because it is responsible for euphoria, physical dependence, and constipation. Unfortunately, a $\mu1$-selective agonist, which produces supraspinal analgesia and sedation, has yet to be identified. Opioids are capable of producing sedation and hypnosis at higher doses but do not cause amnesia. They also activate receptors within the chemoreceptor trigger zone, which can lead to nausea and vomiting. In general, opioids maintain cardiovascular stability, lacking any significant direct myocardial depressant effects. However, bradycardia and hypotension can be noted, likely reflecting a reduction in general sympathetic tone. Dose-dependent respiratory depression is common with opioid administration, as evidenced by a

Table 5 Dexmedetomidine	
Procedural sedation	
IV loading dose	0.5–1 µcg/kg, given slowly over 10 min
IV infusion	0.6 µcg/kg/h (0.2–1 µg/kg/h)
Emergence delirium prevention	
Intranasal	1 µg/kg
IV subanesthetic bolus	0.25 µcg/kg (0.2–0.3 µcg/kg)

decrease in respiratory rate and minute ventilation, despite the increase in tidal volume. Opioids depress the central respiratory drive by inhibiting the medulla's response to hypercarbia and hypoxemia. Higher potency opioids are capable of causing skeletal muscle rigidity when given rapidly, which can impede ventilation without subsequent neuromuscular blockade.

Pharmacokinetics

Morphine is the prototypical opioid agonist and remains the gold standard to which other opioids are compared. However, morphine has several features that may render it less than ideal when compared with hydromorphone. Morphine is relatively hydrophilic, causing a notoriously delayed peak effect ($\sim$15–20 minutes) even when given intravenously. Hydromorphone is quite similar but somewhat easier to titrate because it is more lipophilic, with a faster peak effect ($\sim$5–10 minutes). Both undergo hepatic metabolism; however, morphine is converted into the active byproduct morphine-6-glucuronide metabolites, which hydromorphone lacks.[32] Both agents are renally eliminated with similar elimination half-lives approximating 2 to 4 hours.

The phenylpiperidine opioid subclass, fentanyl, and its congeners, sufentanil, alfentanil, and remifentanil, have pharmacokinetic profiles that may be more ideal for shorter surgical procedures commonly performed in the office-based environment. All of these opioids are more potent than morphine and are quite lipophilic with very rapid onset approximating 30 to 60 seconds and peak effects within 5 minutes. The duration of action, primarily dictated by the redistribution half-life, approximates 30 minutes for fentanyl, 17 minutes for sufentanil, and 14 minutes for alfentanil.[33–35] With the noted exception of remifentanil, all undergo hepatic metabolism to inactive metabolites, such as norfentanyl. Remifentanil is unique because it undergoes metabolism via nonspecific plasma esterases with an extremely rapid terminal half-life approximating 3 to 8 minutes and is devoid of any active metabolites.[36]

Clinical Use

As mentioned previously, these opioid agonists are most frequently used for analgesia during the perioperative period (**Table 6**). All can be titrated to the desired effect, often using the patient's respiratory rate as a rough guide to determine adequate analgesia, with a rate of 10 to 12 breaths per minute being an acceptable target. The extended duration of action of morphine and hydromorphone can be useful when prolonged postoperative analgesia is desired. Clinicians must be certain, however, that the peak effect of any drug administered is verified before dismissal of the patient. The fentanyl congeners can be quite useful for shorter surgical procedures, especially those where adequacy of analgesia can be obtained with local anesthesia. A main benefit of these drugs is their shorter duration of action, which can reduce the risk of complications postoperatively, particularly respiratory depression. Fentanyl, sufentanil, and alfentanil to a lesser degree, can all be given via intermittent boluses, titrated to the desired clinical effect. Remifentanil, because of its rapid metabolic profile, must be administered via continuous infusion to maintain surgical analgesia. In fact, if remifentanil is used, another opioid agonist is recommended to provide postoperative analgesia and to also help combat postoperative hyperalgesia, which can occur with remifentanil.

INHALATIONAL AGENTS (NITROUS OXIDE, VOLATILE AGENTS)

The use of inhalational anesthetic agents for dentistry and oral surgery dates back to the late

Table 6
Opioids

Agent	Route	Dose[a]
		Perioperative Analgesia
Morphine	IV bolus	0.05–0.1 mg/kg
Hydromorphone	IV bolus	0.1–0.2 mg
Fentanyl	IV bolus	1–2 µg/kg
Sufentanil	IV bolus	1–2 µg/kg
Alfentanil	IV bolus	5–15 µg/kg
	Continuous infusion	0.5 µg/kg/min (0.25–1 µg/kg/min)
Remifentanil	Continuous infusion	0.05 µg/kg/min (0.025–0.1 µg/kg/min)

[a] Titrated slowly to effect.

1800s and the time of Horace Wells, William Morton, and Crawford Long[37] and the discovery of modern anesthesia. The first inhalational anesthetic agent was nitrous oxide, followed almost immediately by ether. Although nitrous oxide remains a popular inhalational anesthetic agent, ether has had many successors, the most recent being the fluorinated hydrocarbons isoflurane, sevoflurane, and desflurane.[38] There currently exists no single anesthetic agent that can provide every desired aspect of anesthesia; however, these inhalational agents are in all likelihood the closest, capable of producing hypnosis, analgesia, amnesia, sedation/unconsciousness, and skeletal muscle relaxation.[39,40] In addition, the delivery of these drugs via the inhalational route provides an extremely rapid onset of clinical activity, facilitating easy titration to the desired effect, and a rapid recovery rivaled by few other anesthetic agents.

Pharmacodynamics

Nitrous oxide and the other volatile agents all act to cause global CNS depression; however, the actual mechanism of action by which they produce their clinical effects is yet to be completely understood and identified. Nitrous oxide and the current volatile agents are known to interact with a wide variety of ion channels present within the central and peripheral nervous systems.[38] In addition, nitrous oxide also acts as an opioid receptor agonist as well as an NMDA receptor antagonist, similar to ketamine. The minimum alveolar concentration (MAC) is a useful means to compare the potency of the various agents, with a single MAC being the alveolar concentration in which 50% of patients fail to respond to a surgical stimulus. MAC also allows for estimations of anesthetic depth because MAC values are additive. For example, a patient administered 3% desflurane (~0.5 MAC) plus 50% nitrous oxide/50% oxygen (~0.5 MAC) is receiving roughly 1 MAC total of inhalational anesthetics. Although the volatile agents and nitrous oxide are all associated with dose-dependent depression of the respiratory drive, increases in respiratory rate, and reductions in tidal volume and minute ventilation, the nitrous oxide effects are minimized when it is used alone for minimal sedation. Nitrous oxide does not cause, nor break a bronchospasm, because it lacks the significant bronchodilatory effects noted with the volatile agents, specifically sevoflurane. Volatile gases cause dose-dependent myocardial depression and peripheral vasodilation, manifesting commonly as bradycardia and significant hypotension. In comparison, nitrous oxide is rather benign, causing minimal cardiovascular alterations because of the mild dose-dependent myocardial contractility depression being offset by a modest increase in sympathetic tone. The net result is a rather stable cardiovascular profile in otherwise healthy patients. An additional difference is the potential to trigger malignant hyperthermia, which is present with all volatile agents but completely absent with nitrous oxide.

Pharmacokinetics

As inhaled anesthetics, the uptake, equilibration, and distribution of the volatile agents and nitrous oxide are primarily dictated by the concentration, flow rate, and solubility (blood:gas partition coefficient) of each gas as well as by the cardiac output of the patient (**Table 7**). Once a positive gas gradient is established at the alveolar level in relation to the blood, the gas begins to saturate the blood plasma. The same phenomenon occurs between the blood plasma and the bodily tissues, with the end result given ample time, and stable drug delivery being the establishment of an equilibrium between the anesthetic partial pressures at the alveolar, blood plasma, and tissue (brain) levels. Isoflurane, sevoflurane, desflurane, and nitrous oxide all undergo some degree of metabolism; however, it is to such a miniscule degree that they are essentially considered unchanged when eliminated. These anesthetic agents are exhaled and eliminated via the lungs, in the reverse of the same processes that dictated their initial uptake and distribution.

Clinical Use

Nitrous oxide is administered concurrently with oxygen most commonly via the traditional nasal hood, which is an open system. These systems can easily incorporate the use of other anesthesia monitors, such as capnography or pulse oximetry,

Table 7 Inhalational agents			
		Partition Coefficients	
Agent	**MAC %**	**Blood:Gas**	**Fat:Blood**
Nitrous oxide	104	0.47	2.3
Isoflurane	6	1.4	45
Sevoflurane	2	0.65	48
Desflurane	6	0.42	27
Comments			
MAC awake	0.3%–0.4% (inhaled drug is sole anesthetic maintenance agent)		

to verify the presence of fresh gas exchange and adequacy of oxygenation, respectively. Patient dose-responses generally follow a bell-shaped curve, with hyperresponders at risk of overdose and oversedation. Unconsciousness has been reported even with the "normal" nitrous oxide dose concentrations of 30% to 50%. As such, nitrous oxide is ideally administered incrementally, with careful titration to the desired clinical endpoint, rather than to a set concentration. Nitrous oxide can also be used concurrently with the volatile agents, thereby providing an additive MAC fraction free of significant cardiovascular effects.

Use of the volatile agents requires additional armamentarium and safety protocols beyond those associated with nitrous oxide alone. A vaporizer is needed to safely administer these volatile agents, often via an anesthesia machine with a closed circuit capable of removing carbon dioxide and recycling the remaining gases. Although any of the aforementioned volatile agents are capable of serving as maintenance anesthetic agents, each has its own distinct advantages/disadvantages. Isoflurane is currently quite economical and a viable option for particularly long cases. Its pharmacokinetic profile is slower than the others, which may lead to a slower, albeit smooth emergence and recovery. Desflurane is the least soluble of the volatile agents; therefore, it is not only the least potent but also the least likely to accumulate within the bodily tissues, combined with the fastest emergence and recovery profile. Although it may be the "fastest" of the volatile agents, it is particularly irritating to the airways, which hampers its utility for mask inductions. Sevoflurane is considered by many to be the preferred volatile agent because of its versatility. Although not as "fast" as desflurane, sevoflurane is non-irritating and is quite effective for mask inductions, particularly when combined with nitrous oxide. The use of volatile agents carries the risk of malignant hyperthermia; therefore, appropriate preparation and precautions are necessary, including the immediate availability of dantrolene.

SUMMARY

Oral and maxillofacial surgeons have a variety of anesthetic agents at their disposal that can be used to provide sedation and anesthesia in the ambulatory dental environment. It is critical that the anesthesia provider inherently understands the pharmacokinetics and pharmacodynamics of each anesthetic agent before its use. Furthermore, clinicians should also take into consideration the requirements of the patient and the surgical procedure itself when selecting anesthetic agents to achieve maximal results. Such an approach permits the delivery of an anesthetic plan tailored specifically to each individual patient.

REFERENCES

1. Moore PA. Sedative-hypnotics, antianxiety drugs, and centrally acting muscle relaxants. In: Yagiela JA, Dowd FJ, Neidle EA, editors. Pharmacology and therapeutics for dentistry. 5th edition. St Louis (MO): Elsevier Mosby; 2004. p. 193–218.
2. Robinson DH, Toledo AH. Historical development of modern anesthesia. J Invest Surg 2012;25(3):141–9.
3. Walder B, Tramer MR, Seeck M. Seizure-like phenomena and propofol: a systematic review. Neurology 2002;58(9):1327–32.
4. Butterworth JF, Mackey DC, Wasnick JD. Intravenous anesthetics. Chapter 9. In: Butterworth JF, Mackey DC, Wasnick JD, editors. Morgan & Mikhail's clinical anesthesiology. 5th edition. New York: The McGraw-Hill Companies; 2013. p. 175–88.
5. Dolin SJ. Drugs and pharmacology. In: Padfield NL, editor. Total intravenous anaesthesia. Oxford (United Kingdom): Butterworth-Heinemann; 2000. p. 13–35.
6. Casagrande AM. Propofol for office oral and maxillofacial anesthesia: the case against low-dose ketamine. J Oral Maxillofac Surg 2006;64(4):693–5.
7. Hiraoka H, Yamamoto K, Miyoshi S, et al. Kidneys contribute to the extrahepatic clearance of propofol in humans, but not lungs and brain. Br J Clin Pharmacol 2005;60(2):176–82.
8. Cillo JE Jr. Analysis of propofol and low-dose ketamine admixtures for adult outpatient dentoalveolar surgery: a prospective, randomized, positive-controlled clinical trial. J Oral Maxillofac Surg 2012;70(3):537–46.
9. Murray MJ. Propofol. In: Murray MJ, Harrison BA, Mueller JT, et al, editors. Faust's anesthesiology review. 4th edition. Philadelphia: Elselvier/Saunders; 2015. p. 163–4.
10. Haas DA, Yagiela JA. Agents used in general anesthesia, deep sedation, and conscious sedation. In: Yagiela JA, Dowd FJ, Neidle EA, editors. Pharmacology and therapeutics for dentistry. 5th edition. St Louis (MO): Elsevier Mosby; 2004. p. 287–306.
11. O'Connor S, Zhang YL, Christians U, et al. Remifentanil and propofol undergo separation and layering when mixed in the same syringe for total intravenous anesthesia. Paediatr Anaesth 2016;26(7):703–9.
12. Celesia GG, Chen RC, Bamforth BJ. Effects of ketamine in epilepsy. Neurology 1975;25(2):169–72.
13. Brown RH, Wagner EM. Mechanisms of bronchoprotection by anesthetic induction agents: propofol versus ketamine. Anesthesiology 1999;90(3): 822–8.
14. Haas DA, Harper DG. Ketamine: a review of its pharmacologic properties and use in ambulatory anesthesia. Anesth Prog 1992;39(3):61–8.

15. Domino EF, Domino SE, Smith RE, et al. Ketamine kinetics in unmedicated and diazepam-premedicated subjects. Clin Pharmacol Ther 1984;36(5):645–53.

16. Grant IS, Nimmo WS, Clements JA. Pharmacokinetics and analgesic effects of i.m. and oral ketamine. Br J Anaesth 1981;53(8):805–10.

17. Annetta MG, Iemma D, Garisto C, et al. Ketamine: new indications for an old drug. Curr Drug Targets 2005;6(7):789–94.

18. Panzer O, Moitra V, Sladen RN. Pharmacology of sedative-analgesic agents: dexmedetomidine, remifentanil, ketamine, volatile anesthetics, and the role of peripheral mu antagonists. Crit Care Clin 2009; 25(3):451–69, vii.

19. Hijazi Y, Boulieu R. Contribution of CYP3A4, CYP2B6, and CYP2C9 isoforms to N-demethylation of ketamine in human liver microsomes. Drug Metab Dispos 2002;30(7):853–8.

20. Herd DW, Anderson BJ, Holford NH. Modeling the norketamine metabolite in children and the implications for analgesia. Paediatr Anaesth 2007;17(9): 831–40.

21. Bolze S, Boulieu R. HPLC determination of ketamine, norketamine, and dehydronorketamine in plasma with a high-purity reversed-phase sorbent. Clin Chem 1998;44(3):560–4.

22. Badrinath S, Avramov MN, Shadrick M, et al. The use of a ketamine-propofol combination during monitored anesthesia care. Anesth Analg 2000; 90(4):858–62.

23. Blaise GA. Ketamine. In: Murray MJ, Harrison BA, Mueller JT, et al, editors. Faust's anesthesiology review. 4th edition. Philadelphia: Elselvier/Saunders; 2015. p. 166–7.

24. Lebrun T, Van Elstraete AC, Sandefo I, et al. Lack of a pre-emptive effect of low-dose ketamine on postoperative pain following oral surgery. Can J Anaesth 2006;53(2):146–52.

25. Hadhimane A, Shankariah M, Neswi KV. Pre-emptive analgesia with ketamine for relief of postoperative pain after surgical removal of impacted mandibular third molars. J Maxillofac Oral Surg 2016;15(2): 156–63.

26. Muzyk AJ, Fowler JA, Norwood DK, et al. Role of alpha2-agonists in the treatment of acute alcohol withdrawal. Ann Pharmacother 2011;45(5):649–57.

27. Kamibayashi T, Maze M. Clinical uses of alpha2-adrenergic agonists. Anesthesiology 2000;93(5): 1345–9.

28. Barash PG. Clinical anesthesia. 6th edition. Philadelphia: Wolters Kluwer/Lippincott Williams & Wilkins; 2009.

29. Yuen VM, Hui TW, Irwin MG, et al. A comparison of intranasal dexmedetomidine and oral midazolam for premedication in pediatric anesthesia: a double-blinded randomized controlled trial. Anesth Analg 2008;106(6):1715–21.

30. Larsson PG, Eksborg S, Lonnqvist PA. Incidence of bradycardia at arrival to the operating room after oral or intravenous premedication with clonidine in children. Paediatr Anaesth 2015;25(9):956–62.

31. Gazelka HM, Rho RH. Opioid pharmacology. In: Murray MJ, Harrison BA, Mueller JT, et al, editors. Faust's anesthesiology review. 4th edition. Philadelphia: Elsevier/Saunders; 2015. p. 168–9.

32. Christrup LL. Morphine metabolites. Acta Anaesthesiol Scand 1997;41(1 Pt 2):116–22.

33. Fentanyl Citrate Injection [package insert]. Lake Forest, IL: Hospira, Inc; 2017.

34. Sufentanil Citrate Injection [package insert]. Lake Forest, IL: Akorn, Inc; 2014.

35. Alfentanil HCl Injection [package insert]. Lake Forest, IL 60045: Akorn, Inc; 2013.

36. Glass PSA, Gan TJ, Howell S. A review of the pharmacokinetics and pharmacodynamics of remifentanil. Anesth Analg 1999;89(Supplement):7.

37. Desai MS, Desai SP. Discovery of modern anesthesia: a counterfactual narrative about Crawford W. Long, Horace Wells, Charles T. Jackson, and William T. G. Morton. AANA J 2015;83(6):410–5.

38. Butterworth JF, Mackey DC, Wasnick JD. Inhalation anesthetics. Chapter 8. In: Butterworth JF, Mackey DC, Wasnick JD, editors. Morgan & Mikhail's clinical anesthesiology. 5th edition. New York: The McGraw-Hill Companies; 2013. p. 153–74.

39. Becker DE, Rosenberg M. Nitrous oxide and the inhalation anesthetics. Anesth Prog 2008;55(4): 124–30 [quiz: 131–2].

40. Wilson S, Alcaino EA. Survey on sedation in paediatric dentistry: a global perspective. Int J Paediatr Dent 2011;21(5):321–32.

The Failed Sedation
Solutions for the Oral and Maxillofacial Surgeon

Robert C. Bosack, DDS[a,b,]*

KEYWORDS

- Failed sedation • Complication • Office-based anesthesia • Patient selection

KEY POINTS

- Failed sedation is the inability to satisfactorily complete a planned procedure (with sedation).
- Failed sedation is an inexorably entwined, multifactorial event, which can be due to unsuitable patient, procedure, or facility choices; inappropriate drug selection/dose; adverse drug response; and/or lack of a shared, structured, and realistic anesthetic plan.
- The true incidence of failed sedation in the oral and maxillofacial surgery office is unknown, but can approach *1 case per month*.
- Failed sedation can best be prevented by communication and realistic alignment of patient expectations.
- Management of failed sedation will most often include lightening anesthetic depth and/or aborting the planned procedure, with patient safety remaining the top priority.

INTRODUCTION AND DEFINITION

Open airway office "anesthesia" can be typically characterized as moderate to deep sedation (with occasional descent into general anesthesia) combined with local anesthesia, with a retreat to moderate sedation for longer cases.[1] Anesthetic protocols in the oral and maxillofacial surgery office routinely include intravenous midazolam and fentanyl, often supplemented with ketamine, nitrous oxide, and/or incremental small propofol boluses. Oral premedication with a benzodiazepine or alpha-2 agonist is sporadically entertained. The 3-fold purpose of these medications is to (1) permit, facilitate, and expedite painful or threatening procedures by blocking pain, and decreasing or eliminating perception; (2) mitigate physical and emotional reactions to painful stimuli; and (3) improve patient satisfaction. These three objectives are best accomplished by providing safe, reversible, drug-induced analgesia, amnesia, anxiolysis, and behavior control in a "stress minimized" setting.[2] Sedation success can be loosely defined as the ability to safely complete the intended procedure, while minimizing pain, anxiety, recall, and the neuroendocrine stress (fight or flight) response (**Box 1**), *and maintain patient satisfaction*. The *event* of inability to successfully complete the planned procedure, to the satisfaction (expectation) of the provider and/or patient/guardian, is termed *failed sedation*. Failed sedation could also include patient combativeness, the (unplanned) use of physical restraint, unexpected postanesthetic recall of intraoperative awareness, and adverse drug effects (benzodiazepine disinhibition and ketamine delirium). "Bad anesthesia begets bad surgery" (Robert Campbell,

Disclosure Statement: The author has nothing to disclose.
[a] Private Practice, 16011 South 108th Avenue, Orland Park, IL 60467, USA; [b] University of Illinois at Chicago College of Dentistry, 801 S. Paulina, Chicago, IL 60612, USA
* Corresponding author. 16011 South 108th Avenue, Orland Park, IL 60467.
E-mail address: r.bosack@comcast.net

Oral Maxillofacial Surg Clin N Am 30 (2018) 165–169
https://doi.org/10.1016/j.coms.2018.01.004

DDS, personal communication, 2015). Compromised surgery includes torn flaps, damage to adjacent structures, and so forth. For purposes of this discussion, failed sedation will not include complications of anesthesia, such as adverse cardiac and pulmonary responses, nausea, vomiting, pulmonary soiling, and myocardial ischemia, among others. Certainly, however, anesthetic complications cannot be isolated from failed sedations.

CAUSE AND SPECTRUM OF FAILED SEDATION

Failed sedation is a multifactorial event that can be due to and compounded by suboptimal (1) drug choices, doses, adverse side effects, and/or technique; (2) patient selection, preparation, and drug responses; and (3) surgical case selection. Practitioner training, experience, preparation, ability, and willingness to progress to general anesthesia can also play a role in inability to successfully complete a planned procedure.

Drug choices and anesthetic technique play a large role in the success or failure of sedation in the oral and maxillofacial surgery office. It is useful to recall the definition of deep sedation/analgesia, which is a drug-induced depression of consciousness during which patients cannot be easily aroused but respond purposefully following repeated or painful stimuli and general anesthesia, where patients are unarousable. Therefore, when in a state of deep sedation, if local anesthesia is inadequate, or if systemic analgesia is inadequate, one would anticipate patient arousal, movement (combativeness), increases in blood pressure and heart rate, and so forth: the neuroendocrine sympathetic stress response. Many would interpret this as failed sedation. The most obvious scenario for this circumstance is not waiting for administered drugs to take full effect, or rushing the medication. Possible strategies for remediation include waiting for drug action, ensuring profound local anesthesia, redosing or introducing alternative drugs, progression to full general anesthesia (an attendant side effects), or sedation/case abandonment.

Two other "failed sedation" scenarios deserve mention. A one-drug, benzodiazepine regimen can, at times, prove to be less than satisfactory to obtund perception and reaction to the administration of local anesthesia, and can, in fact, increase cold, heat, and electrical pain perception.[3] Finally, stage II excitement (between deep sedation and general anesthesia) can occasionally be experienced, with attendant patient movement and adverse physiologic changes interfering with case completion.

Ketamine delirium[4] is not always predictable, but may be predisposed at higher doses, in adolescent female patients, and in those with psychiatric illness. Because there is no reversal for ketamine, management includes minimizing external visual, auditory, and tactile stimulation and waiting for drug redistribution and elimination. Paradoxic benzodiazepine disinhibition (psychomotor and cognitive dysfunction) is also a possibility that tends to occur in younger patients, perhaps seen more often in those who struggle to internalize their pre–sedation anxiety (impulse control). Treatment options include benzodiazepine reversal, use of other agents, or waiting for drug diffusion away from central receptors. Benzodiazepine redosing is rarely successful in this instance. Nelson and colleagues[5] concluded that sedation outcome was significantly associated with high scores over the temperament domains of effortful control, attention focusing, and inhibitory control, as determined by a questionnaire. However, this begs the question that successful attempts at sedation would exclude those very patients who might benefit the most from it.

Anesthetic technique depends not only on drug choices but also on real-time, robust, moment by moment monitoring of drug effect.[6] Intense monitoring oftentimes will provide not only a window of safety but also invite possibilities of alternative drug strategies, as interventions become proactive rather than reactive. Similarly, rapid detection of adversity can limit the duration and severity of adverse side effects, minimizing their contribution to failed sedation.

Patient selection and responses to anesthetic drugs can also contribute to failed sedation. Virtually all anesthetic drugs have adverse side effects, which include not only disinhibition and delirium but also loss of upper airway tone, ventilatory depression, and adverse cardiovascular changes. The appearance of these side effects will limit both choices and doses of anesthetic drugs, which can prove to be necessary for successful sedation. In these types of cases, "healthier" patients are often better suited to *tolerate* adverse cardiopulmonary challenges and are more likely able to *compensate* for these challenges. In both instances, the likelihood of a successful sedation increases. Resilient patients are better able to tolerate hypoxemia, hypotension, and tachycardia; these include patients receiving supplemental oxygen, patients with relatively large functional residual capacities, patients with patent coronary vessels, and patients who are adequately hydrated. Patients who have physiologic and anatomic reserve can call on those reserves to compensate for the physiologic demands of anesthesia and surgery. Patients with adequate reserves include those who can mount a sympathetic response to hypotension (ie, those not on opioids or beta-blockers), those who can maintain ventilation (lower doses of ventilatory depressant opioids), and those who have full airway patency and function (ie, those who do not have large necks and those who do not snore). As such, sedation failure can be more likely in patients listed in **Box 2**.

Patient preparation is the most important predictor of sedation success. The adoption and agreement of a shared, structured anesthetic plan is paramount. Open, honest, and unrushed communication will properly align patient expectations and predict sedation success. An obvious example would be the patient with severe obstructive sleep apnea who insists on "not waking up in the middle" of the planned procedure. This request would represent an unachievable goal for a practitioner practicing open airway anesthesia. In this case, treatment at an outside facility to protect and manage the difficult airway would be more appropriate. Otherwise, the anticipated problem should be shared with the patient, who then

"learns to own their disease." In this instance, patient becomes engaged in his or her treatment and may be better able to understand and accept limitations to their desires, as expectations become appropriately aligned.

Appropriate case selection can be predictive of sedation success. Choosing procedures that can be performed with local anesthesia only will increase the success of sedation, when needed for anxiolysis and amnesia. Contrarily, procedures involving regions not readily amenable to local anesthesia, for example, deeper procedures involving the floor of the mouth, inferior border of the mandible, or superior regions of the maxilla, can be difficult to complete with sedation only, as profound local anesthesia can be difficult to attain in these regions.

INCIDENCE

As noted above, the extreme variability of definitions and thresholds of both patient and provider, combined with the lack of reporting and databases, hampers the ability to accurately identify the incidence of failed sedation. Lack of oversight and peer review, coupled with often absent administrative mechanisms for identifying and reporting quality of care, makes the incidence of failed sedation largely unknown.[7] Likewise, the literature remains sparse regarding failed sedation. Senel and colleagues[8] reported a 1% to 2% incidence for ambulatory patients in oral and maxillofacial surgery practices, which could represent *one or more cases per month* in a busy practice. Like all adverse, but rare events, statistical power will remain insufficient. As such, each circumstance of failed sedation deserves maximal attention. The World Wide Web is replete with "horror stories" of patients "being awake" during their surgery.

PREVENTION

Strategies to minimize or prevent failed sedations are summarized in **Box 3**.

Appropriate patient selection has been addressed earlier, emphasizing the selection

---

Box 2
Patient characteristics that can predispose failed sedation

- Upper airway "challenges"
- Extremes of age
- Disorders of habitus/feeding
- Cancer, cancer treatment
- Disordered breathing during sleep
- > ASA Physical Status II
- Lack of a shared anesthetic plan

Box 3
Strategies to minimize failed sedation

- Appropriate patient selection
- Realistic patient expectations
- Appropriate case selection
- Adequate pain control
- Realistic acceptance of provider limitations

of "healthier" patients, who are better able to tolerate and compensate for physiologic changes associated with the neuroendocrine stress response. Similarly, practitioners who take the time to appropriately align patient expectations better position themselves for successful completion of planned procedures.

Unless general anesthesia is planned, *adequate pain (and anxiety) control* is mandatory. Profound local anesthesia is paramount. Well-targeted injections and allowing adequate time for nerve penetration are cornerstones of good anesthetic technique. The use of either buffered local anesthetic or local anesthetic without vasoconstrictor will hasten onset and may enhance the profundity of anesthesia, because acidic vasoconstrictors, which reduce the lipid-soluble moiety needed to penetrate nerve tissue, is not present. Allowing adequate time for sedative drug action (not rushing the drugs) also adds to the likelihood of sedation success. Drug responses for individual patients lie on the standard distribution curve (**Fig 1**), which means that in at least one-third of all cases, patients will either hyperrespond or hyporespond, and that sometimes the full clinical onset of drugs such as intravenous midazolam and fentanyl can take up to 10 minutes or more. Preanesthetic anxiety control is best achieved with patient rapport, a stress-minimized environment, and possible use of oral premedication.

MANAGEMENT

There are 3 strategies to manage failed sedations, once identified and accepted. Patient safety assumes upmost priority at all times.

An attractive option, which is often subconsciously entertained and readily executed, is the addition of increased dose or alternative drugs to *deepen the level of anesthesia*. Two potential problems can arise in this circumstance. As depth of anesthesia increases, so does the appearance of adverse side effects, such as loss of upper airway tone and patency, ventilatory depression, and adverse cardiovascular changes (the procedure becomes victim of its own success). All 3 of these adversities can occur suddenly, without warning and at unexpected doses, because patients can rapidly transition between moderate and deep sedation and general anesthesia. The second problem involves the unnoticed (and underappreciated) accumulation of drugs in fat and muscle stores, such as midazolam and fentanyl, the initial effect of which is terminated by redistribution *away from central receptors*. In this instance, redistribution of drugs *from fat and muscle stores* can once again lead to prolonged and exaggerated clinical effects. In both cases, a deeper than intended depth of anesthesia can present challenges to the unsuspecting clinician.

At the other end of the spectrum, early *abandonment of sedation*, with the intention of completing the anticipated procedure under local anesthesia only or residual light sedation, remains a possibility. Patient outcomes and attitudes remain a variable here; certainly, preprocedural patient rapport becomes most advantageous. In the relative absence of anxiolysis and analgesia, adequate local anesthesia is mandatory to minimize the neuroendocrine stress response.

Abandonment of both sedation and surgery must remain both an option and a priority when patient safety is compromised. In this case, location of service and possibly the provider is changed.

SUMMARY

The tremendous growth in office-based sedation in oral and maxillofacial surgery brings with it challenges for successful completion of surgical procedures with sedation. It is clear from this discussion that it is impossible to successfully sedate all patients. Choosing the right drug and dose regimen can be challenging, especially in patients who are naïve to anesthesia. Underdosing can lead to pain perception, patient movement and combativeness, awareness with recall, and the sympathetic neuroendocrine stress response. Overdosing can lead to unintended loss of upper airway tone, hypoventilation/apnea, adverse cardiovascular changes, and prolonged sedation (with its attendant problems). Adverse drug reactions cannot always be predicted. In many instances, once "anesthetic control" is lost, it is difficult, if not impossible, to regain, as "chasing pain" is rarely successful, without progression to stage III anesthesia.

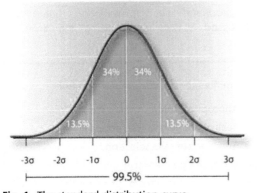

Fig. 1. The standard distribution curve.

REFERENCES

1. Fain DW, Ferguson BL, Indresano AT, et al. The oral and maxillofacial surgery team model. J Oral Maxillofac Surg 2017;75:1097–100.

2. Stevens RL, Reed KL. Failed sedation. In: Bosack RC, Lieblich S, editors. Anesthesia complications in the dental office. Ames (IA): Wiley Blackwell; 2014. p. 201–5.

3. Frolich MA, Zhang K, Ness T. Effect of sedation on pain perception. Anesthesiology 2013;118:611–21.

4. Platt CW. Beneath the furrowed brow: a ketamine journey in the ER. Anesthesiology 2016;125:599–601.

5. Nelson TM, Griffith TM, Lane KJ, et al. Temperament as a predictor of nitrous oxide inhalation sedation success. Anesth Prog 2017;64:17–21.

6. Bosack RC. Monitoring for the oral and maxillofacial surgeon. Oral Maxillofac Surg Clin North Am 2017; 29:159–68.

7. Quattrone MS. Is the physician office the wild, wild west of health care? J Ambul Care Manage 2000; 23:64–73.

8. Senel AC, Altintas NY, Senel FC, et al. Evaluation of sedation in oral and maxillofacial surgery in ambulatory patients: failure and complications. Oral Surg Oral Med Oral Pathol Oral Radiol 2012;114:592–6.

Anesthesia for the Pediatric Oral and Maxillofacial Surgery Patient

Deepak G. Krishnan, DDS

KEYWORDS

- Pediatric anesthesia • Training standards in pediatric anesthesia for OMS
- Techniques in pediatric anesthesia

KEY POINTS

- Anatomy and physiology as it relates to pediatric anesthesia is described.
- Current training standards for oral and maxillofacial surgeons in pediatric anesthesia are outlined.
- NPO guidelines for pediatric patients are presented.
- Anesthetic techniques and monitoring for pediatric anesthesia are considered.
- Anesthetic considerations for children with autism spectrum disorders and for children with attention deficit hyperactivity disorder.

INTRODUCTION

Children are not small adults and should never be taken for granted as such while planning administration of pediatric anesthesia in the oral and maxillofacial surgeon (OMS) office. Although OMSs may be astutely familiar and expertly talented in providing anesthesia for adults in their offices, it would not be prudent to apply the same confidence to anesthetizing children outside the operating rooms. The pediatric patient exhibits stark contrasts in their behavioral psychology, anatomy, and physiology, and those differences must be respected when providing anesthesia in this age group. The intent of this article is to identify key anatomic and physiologic differences in the pediatric population and address some common techniques in the safe practice of pediatric ambulatory anesthesia.

ANATOMY AND PHYSIOLOGY

The American Academy of Pediatrics and bodies such as the US Food and Drug Administration define pediatric subpopulations[1] as shown in **Table 1**.

Airway Anatomy and Pulmonary Physiology in Children

Younger children have disproportionately large heads perched on their tiny necks, connected to a wide thorax of immature cartilaginous ribs atop a large protuberant abdomen. Both tongue and tonsils are also disproportionately large, relative to the size of adjacent anatomy. Additionally, they have small nasal passages and are obligate nasal breathers until they are about 5 months of age.

The geometry of the pediatric airway was long considered to be an arrangement of the cartilaginous and other soft tissue structures in the neck to form a funnel shape. The long floppy epiglottis and an anterior and more cephalad larynx are major differences in the airway anatomy of a child and an adult. The shorter neck of a child makes the position of the larynx at the level of C4, whereas it is

Disclosure Statement: The author has nothing to disclose.
Division of Oral Maxillofacial Surgery, Department of Surgery, University of Cincinnati, Cincinnati, OH 45242, USA
E-mail address: deepak.krishnan@uc.edu

Oral Maxillofacial Surg Clin N Am 30 (2018) 171–181
https://doi.org/10.1016/j.coms.2018.02.002
1042-3699/18/© 2018 Elsevier Inc. All rights reserved.

Table 1	
Age-based definitions of pediatric patients	
Pediatric Subpopulation	**Approximate Age Range**
Newborn	Birth to 1 mo of age
Infant	1 mo to 2 y of age
Child	2 to 12 y of age
Adolescent	12 to 21 y of age

Table 2		
Comparison of pulmonary physiologic parameters of the child versus the adult		
Variable	**Infant**	**Adult**
Respiratory frequency	30–50	12–16
Tidal volume (mL/kg)	6–8	7
Dead space (mL/kg)	2–2.5	2.2
Function reserve capacity (mL/kg)	25	40
Oxygen consumption (mL/kg/min)	6–8	3–4

much lower in an adult at the level of C6. The notion that the pediatric airway is funnel shaped has been challenged in recently studies involving computed tomography scans of neonates and infants.[2] These studies have suggested that the pediatric airway is an elliptical structure with the subglottic area being the narrowest portion of the ellipse. The elliptical shape is particularly prominent between the subglottic region and the cricoid. Additionally, these studies have shown that the airway is wider anteroposteriorly and narrows in the transverse dimension from the subglottic region to the cricoid. The older the child, the more these airways start assuming the shape of the previously described cone. A previous study by the same group suggested that the subglottic area is the narrowest transversely, and that it is the most likely area of resistance to the passage of an endotracheal tube rather than the area of the cricoid.[3]

There are significant differences in the pulmonary anatomy and physiology in children. Their ribs are more cartilaginous in their composition and more horizontal in their arrangement when compared with adults. This factor increases their chest wall compliance, making them more prone to chest wall collapse during inspiration, and leaves them with low residual lung volumes on expiration. Their lung architecture is characterized by alveoli that are smaller in size and fewer in number. The intercostal muscles and diaphragmatic musculature are weaker. Because the rapidly growing child has increased oxygen consumption, their limited physiologic reserve renders them less able to tolerate hypoxemia, and they desaturate more rapidly and have short safe apnea times Children compensate for the lower volume and reserve by increasing respiratory rate. As such, minute ventilation (tidal volume × breaths per minute) can only be maintained by increasing the respiratory rate. This factor is demonstrated by the finding that the respiratory rate is almost double that of an adult, at any given level of activity (**Table 2**).

Upper respiratory tract infections (URIs) are common occurrences in children of school age. There is ample evidence to suggest that the increased airway reactivity in children with URIs make them more susceptible to increased risk of respiratory complications under anesthesia. Scientific literature on the topic provides a range of information. For the clinician looking to answer a simple question, "Should we anesthetize a child with a recent mild-moderate URI?", it can sometimes be challenging to distill the data available. There are no case-controlled studies available and almost all of the available information is based on retrospective observational studies. There is some evidence of this type that suggests that children with a mild URI may be safely anesthetized because the problems encountered are generally easily treated without long-term sequelae. Most credible data on this topic also are in the context of airway instrumentation—supraglottic airway or intubation being involved in the anesthetic technique. A recent prospectively conducted study showed that children with URI did worse when a laryngeal mask airway was placed.[4] So, is an OMS who performs a quick and simple procedure in the office with anxiolysis and a nonintubated airway safer while anesthetizing a child with a mild URI? There is no evidence that suggests evidence to prove or disprove that scenario.

When in doubt, postponing the case until the child is well is probably the prudent approach.

Cardiovascular Anatomy and Physiology in Children

Younger children have a relatively noncompliant and fixed left ventricle. The size of their heart and vasculature increase with age. The limited mobility of the left side of the heart limits diastolic fill and, therefore, the stroke volume. Because cardiac output depends on heart rate and stroke volume, an inherent decrease in stroke volume suggests that the heart rate must increase to maintain cardiac output. Both systolic and diastolic pressures increase with age and increased size of organs (**Table 3**).

Table 3
Age-related changes in cardiovascular parameters of the pediatric patient

Age	Heart Rate (bpm)	Systolic Blood Pressure (mm Hg)	Diastolic Blood Pressure (mm Hg)
Newborn	110–150	60–75	27
6 mo	80–150	95	45
2 y	85–125	95	50
4 y	75–115	98	57
8 y	60–110	112	60

The immature autonomic nervous system of younger patients blunts their reflex ability to respond to hypotension, via either tachycardia or vasoconstriction. A decreased response to exogenous catecholamines can also be anticipated. Neonates and infants respond to loss of volume by being hypotensive and are rarely tachycardic.

Cardiac arrest in otherwise healthy children is rarely due to true cardiac events. It is almost always pulmonary driven and is a response to hypoxic insults. Hypoxia and respiratory embarrassments trigger bradycardia, hypotension, and, eventually, asystole in children. This is particularly pertinent to the sedated child with potential airway compromise in the OMS office.

The renal and gastrointestinal systems in the pediatric population also deserves mention. Normal kidney function is not reached until a child is approximately 2 years of age. Even older children undergoing anesthesia in the office require meticulous and appropriate fluid administration and dosing of medications.

Summary of Pediatric Anatomy and Physiology

The pediatric airway is more susceptible to obstruction owing to its size and anatomic position. Airway obstruction and respiratory events cause hypoxia quicker in children owing to lack of resilience and reserve. Hypoxia will usually lead to bradycardia, owing to parasympathetic excess. This often leads to hypotension, because cardiac output is heart rate variable in a fixed stroke volume heart. Bradycardia will result in asystole without early and successful remediation.

CURRENT TRAINING STANDARDS FOR ORAL AND MAXILLOFACIAL SURGEONS IN PEDIATRIC ANESTHESIA

The standards mandated by the Commission on Dental Accreditation specify training in pediatric anesthesia to OMS residents.[5] Currently, the standards that pertain to pediatric anesthesia are standards 4-3.1, 4-9, and 4-9.1.

Standard 4-3.1 states: Anesthesia Service: The assignment must be for a minimum of 5 months, should be consecutive and one of these months should be dedicated to pediatric anesthesia. The resident must function as an anesthesia resident with commensurate level of responsibility.

Standard 4.9 states: The off-service rotation in anesthesia must be supplemented by longitudinal and progressive experience throughout the training program in all aspects of pain and anxiety control. The outpatient surgery experience must ensure adequate training to competence in general anesthesia/deep sedation for oral and maxillofacial surgery procedures, including competence in airway management, on adult and pediatric patients.

Standard 4-9.1 states, The cumulative anesthetic experience of each graduating resident must include administration of general anesthesia/deep sedation to a minimum of 300 patients. A minimum of 150 of these cases must be ambulatory anesthetics for oral and maxillofacial surgery. A minimum of 50 of the 300 patients must be pediatric (18 years of age or younger).

The document specifies that "a pediatric anesthesia patient is defined as 18 years of age or younger."

At the time of preparing this article, the Committee on Education and Training of the American Association of Oral Maxillofacial Surgeons is in the process of recommending some key changes to these standards.

The ability to control anxiety and pain, and to provide anesthesia for our pediatric population is a task that is taken seriously by our training programs. Although minimal numbers do not necessarily ensure competency, they are a definitely a way to guarantee uniform exposure of our trainees to methods to assess the pediatric airway and physiology, and to teach techniques in pediatric anesthesia.

CURRENT EQUIPMENT, PERSONNEL, AND MONITORING GUIDELINES

The optimum care of the pediatric patient under anesthesia in the nonoperating room setting, especially in the OMS office, is guided by several entities.

State and local guidelines may vary as to the recommendations regarding qualification of personnel present during pediatric anesthesia in the OMS office. In general, pediatric advanced life support certification is recommended for key personnel. Although the literature is largely silent on the scientific basis of recommendations and guidelines as it pertains to the ideal number of personnel caring for the child under anesthesia in the nonoperating room setting, it is generally accepted that deeper levels of anesthesia require dedicated monitoring personnel and additional trained hands responsible for the welfare of this child. All personnel are expected to be aware and trained in management of an emergency, should one arise. Pediatric advanced life support protocols standardize responses in the event of an emergency resuscitation.

The American Association of Oral Maxillofacial Surgeons Parameters of Care on Anesthesia[6] states that, although

[A]rrests are rare events, and in the anxiety of a pediatric resuscitation the calculation of quickly needed emergency drugs may be particularly challenging. One-page printouts of dosages in milliliters for the known concentrations of the commonly used drugs that would be required for the actual weight of the particular pediatric patient being anesthetized can facilitate a smooth, coordinated, and most likely successful resuscitation.

Multiple references are available for determining pediatric dosages such as the Broselow Tape, smart phone apps, and a download available from the American Dental Society of Anesthesia.

In general, the American Society of Anesthesiologists (ASA) Practice Recommendations for Pediatric Anesthesia recommends specialized pediatric equipment be readily available. This includes airway equipment for all ages of pediatric patients including ventilation masks, laryngeal mask airways, endotracheal tubes, oral and nasopharyngeal airways, and laryngoscopes with pediatric blades.

Further, a mechanism to provide positive-pressure ventilation appropriate for infants and children must be available, as should intravenous (IV) fluid administration equipment, including pediatric volumetric fluid administration devices, intravascular catheters in all pediatric sizes, and devices for intraosseous fluid administration.

Regardless of the level of anesthesia provided, standard ASA monitoring is recommended, and includes noninvasive size-appropriate monitoring equipment for the measurement of blood pressure, pulse oximetry, capnography, anesthetic gas concentrations, inhaled oxygen concentration, electrocardiography, and temperature as per ASA standards as well as a pediatric precordial stethoscope bell.

Additionally, a resuscitation cart should be stocked with equipment appropriate for pediatric patients of all ages seen in the practice, including pediatric defibrillator paddles and vasoactive resuscitative medications in appropriate pediatric concentrations. Facilities that provide inhalational anesthesia should be prepared with dantrolene sodium and measures to respond to possible malignant hyperthermia (MH) events. Specialized equipment for the management of the difficult pediatric airway by a variety of techniques for airway control, intubation, and ventilation, including but not limited to specialized intubating devices, supraglottic airways, and emergency cricothyrotomy sets, should be stocked and frequently checked during emergency drills and maintained.

A new set of preoperative vital signs, including weight of the child and a focused airway examination before the procedure that includes visualization of the airway and auscultation of the heart and lungs are recommended. Particular attention should be given to the tonsillar size because tonsillar hypertrophy can be an important component of the airway examination. The Fishbaugh classification is used by many to describe tonsillar size. Documentation of these findings should be a part of the anesthesia record.

The anesthesia record itself is a time-oriented anesthesia document with the following components:

Anesthetic agents, including dosages, routes of administration, and times of administration.
Continuous monitoring including heart rate, blood pressure, ventilation, arterial oxygen saturation, end-tidal carbon dioxide, and temperature (when indicated) on at least a 5-minute interval; and
Continuous electrocardiographic monitoring.

NPO GUIDELINES

An Updated Report by the American Society of Anesthesiologists Task Force on Preoperative Fasting and the Use of Pharmacologic Agents to Reduce the Risk of Pulmonary Aspiration published in 2017[7] makes the following recommendations. The guidelines emphasize identifying those patients at increased risk of pulmonary aspiration, namely, those who are obese, have diabetes, and so on. Children in general have a higher incidence of reflux and must be taken into consideration while suggesting NPO orders before planned procedures.

Recommendations for Clear Liquids

Clear liquids may be ingested for up to 2 hours before procedures requiring general anesthesia, regional anesthesia, or procedural sedation and analgesia.

Preoperative Fasting of Breast Milk

For healthy neonates (<44 gestational weeks) and infants, fasting from the intake of breast milk for 4 or more hours before elective procedures requiring general anesthesia, regional anesthesia, or procedural sedation and analgesia should be maintained.

Preoperative Fasting of Infant Formula

Infant formula may be ingested for up to 6 hours before elective procedures requiring general anesthesia, regional anesthesia, or procedural sedation and analgesia.

Preoperative Fasting of Solids and Nonhuman Milk

A light meal or nonhuman milk may be ingested for up to 6 hours before elective procedures requiring general anesthesia, regional anesthesia, or procedural sedation and analgesia. Additional fasting time (eg, ≥8 hours) may be needed in cases of patient intake of fried foods, fatty foods, or meat. Consider both the amount and type of foods ingested when determining an appropriate fasting period. Because nonhuman milk is similar to solids in gastric emptying time, consider the amount ingested when determining an appropriate fasting period.

There are currently no separate recommendations for the pediatric population as it relates to the use of preoperative pharmacologic agents for prevention of pulmonary aspiration including gastrointestinal stimulants, antiemetics, anticholinergics, and antacids. As per the guidelines, offering clear liquids[a] up to 2 hours before induction decreases hunger and irritability in the child, keeps them hydrated, and minimizes challenges in starting a peripheral IV line and decreases hypoglycemia.

PEDIATRIC ANESTHESIA TECHNIQUES
Alleviating Anxiety: Premedication in the Pediatric Population

The primary objective of using premedication in (adult or) pediatric patient is to reduce anxiety and allow acceptance or a mask or an IV to proceed with an anesthetic to the next level. A large majority of children are anxious at the appointment for a procedure in the OMS office. An increased sympathetic tone from this anxiety now makes induction and maintenance of anesthesia more challenging. Anxious patients are 3 times more likely to miss appointments and often require more hand-holding and chair time. Despite the best efforts of the anesthesia team, an unpleasant experience leaves enduring memories for the child and parents and may negatively impact future experiences. The idea of a premedication thus becomes appealing to not only reduce anxiety to "show" for the appointment, but also allows the team to move forward with the anesthetic and surgical plan in a child who is conscious, cooperative, and comfortable.

Premedication can be administered via enteral (oral), parenteral (often intramuscular [IM]), and inhalational routes. Although the enteral route is the least threatening and most convenient way to administer premedication, it has several disadvantages. It primarily relies on the cooperation of the child (and the parent). The dosing is often empirical and the drug cannot be truly titrated. There is a variable response and an equally unpredictable recovery pattern to oral premedication. The often unpredictable and extended times of action of medication may hinder treatment plans on a busy procedure day. Oral predication is often flavored for acceptance by a child and can be available in a variety of creative forms Including syrups, popsicles, and lozenges. Nasal sprays are less well-tolerated by children. An ideal premedication should of course be rapidly absorbed, must then have a rapid onset of action with a high therapeutic index, and should not delay recovery. Various medications including benzodiazepines, histamine blockers, opioids, scopolamine, barbiturates, and alpha agonists (dexmedetomidine and clonidine) have been used as premedication.

Several factors, including ease of absorption and limited cardiovascular effects, make benzodiazepines a desirable choice. Drugs in this class commonly used as premedication includes

---

[a]Clear fluids are limited to water, apple juice, black coffee without milk cream or creamer, clear tea, Gatorade, infant electrolyte solutions (Pedialyte), and clear carbonated beverages.

diazepam, triazolam, and midazolam. Oral midazolam in a liquid form is well-tolerated by children. These 3 medications have some characteristic differences (**Table 4**).

Diazepam has had a long history of use and has been proven to reduce preoperative anxiety and is well-studied in the pediatric population for its efficacy and safety. It has proven to not delay discharge. In very young patients, it is safer to administer it in the office even as a premedication because of its effects on postural stability.

Oral midazolam has a rapid onset of action, short duration of action, leaves no active metabolites, and has the desirable effect of retrograde amnesia. It is available as pleasantly flavored syrups and popsicles, and is easily accepted by the child. The dosing recommended for premedication is 0.5 to 1.0 mg/kg with a 15- to 20-mg maximum dose. This dose is expected to be effective for approximately 30 minutes. This oral dose should not affect heart rate, respiratory rate, or blood pressure significantly. The major disadvantages of this drug is that it does not provide any analgesic effects. Furthermore, 3% to 4% of children can have paradoxic responses to midazolam causing dysphoria, blurred vision, and undesirable behavior. Like all other oral premedications, oral midazolam also may be difficult to titrate, may have unreliable absorption, and moderate failure rates. Other medications such as triazolam have not been well-studied in children.

Dexmedetomidine is gaining popularity as a single agent sedative for MRI or simple procedures. It is an alpha$_2$ agonist and not a GABA-mimetic drug like benzodiazepines or propofol. Its significant advantage is that the sedation it provides mimics natural sleep, anxiolysis, analgesia, sympatholysis, with minimal respiratory depression. The current recommended dose for premedication purposes are 3 to 4 µg/kg intranasal and 1 to 4 µg/kg dosing orally.

Ketamine is another drug that can be used for oral premedication. The dose recommended is 6 mg/kg. At this dose, it typically takes 20 minutes to onset and can provide sedation lasting up to 30 minutes.

Parenteral Routes of Anesthesia

Intramuscular anesthesia technique

The greatest advantage of this route of administration of anesthesia is a certain predictability of onset of anesthesia, even for the most uncooperative of children. The disadvantage is that the rapidity of the onset of anesthesia depends on the drug used and the site of injection, and that it has the potential to be an unpleasant experience for a cooperative child. Many medications including benzodiazepines, ketamine, and dexmedetomidine have been used in the IM technique.

Ketamine seems to be the more commonly choice of OMSs using this route. Ketamine is a drug that is a potent analgesic and amnesic that is known to dissociate the cortical and limbic system, thus disrupting the interpretation of visual, auditory, and painful stimuli. It provides what is referred to as dissociative anesthesia. In subanesthetic doses, it can provide analgesia without respiratory depression and can reduces narcotic requirements. The recommended IM dose of ketamine is 3 to 4 mg/kg. Practitioners often add a benzodiazepine such as midazolam and glycopyrrolate to the same syringe as the ketamine to enhance its action and reduce some of the undesired side effects. Ketamine can cause increased salivation, heart rate, blood pressure, and intracranial pressures. It stimulates smooth muscle dilatation, which reduces the risk of bronchospasm. It is important to note that ketamine comes in 2 concentrations, 50 mg/mL and 100 mg/mL. The higher concentration is desirable for IM injection to minimize volume at the injection site. For larger children, the lower concentration can result in injection volumes that exceed 3 mL, which is not recommended for a single site.

A phenomenon called emergence delirium is associated with the use of ketamine that makes practitioners wary of this drug. The concomitant use of benzodiazepines or propofol can reduce the risk of ketamine-induced delirium. The following have been identified as risk factors for emergence delirium with the use of ketamine:

- Female gender;
- Age greater than 10 years;
- Underlying psychiatric disorder;
- IV route;
- High dose; and
- Excessive noise stimulation upon emergence.

Table 4
Comparison of diazepam, triazolam, and midazolam

Drug	Onset	Elimination
Diazepam	Rapid	Slow
Triazolam	Intermediate	Very rapid
Midazolam	Very rapid	Rapid

The IM technique requires preparing the parent and the staff for IM injection, especially in the uncooperative child; a quiet room with minimal stimuli and provision of enough time on the schedule for the onset of action of anesthesia is ideal for this technique. Monitors must be placed as soon as the child becomes cooperative and should remain in place until discharge. Preparation to escalate to another route of administration of the anesthetic or redosing IM route can be helpful. Longer recovery times can be anticipated with higher preoperative IM dosages.

Intravenous anesthetic technique

The IV route remains the most predictable route of administration of both anesthetic and resuscitation medications. It offers the advantage of rapidity of onset and offset of medications. It does require the placement of a catheter in a peripheral vein, which can be challenging in pediatric patients. Meticulous administration of both the drugs and the fluids require that size appropriate equipment be available, as discussed earlier. Preoperative calculation of drug doses both for anesthesia and emergencies is mandatory. Many apps available on mobile devices and dosing calculators are available on the Internet for accuracy.

Drugs such as benzodiazepines, opioids, ketamine, and propofol remain the mainstay in pediatric IV anesthesia in weight appropriate doses. Single drugs or combinations of these medications provide appropriate environment to perform a procedure achieving the desired goals of anxiolysis, amnesia, analgesia, immobilization, sedation, and hypnosis. The IV route provides safety, rapid onset, rapid offset, and predictable recovery. The IV catheter is recommended to be maintained until discharge and the recovery areas need to be equipped with IV/IO equipment in case of premature loss of this angiocatheter.

Using an infusion pump for longer procedures minimize fluctuations in drug serum concentrations, ensuring a smoother intraoperative anesthetic course. Typically, the pump ensures enhanced cardiovascular and respiratory stability, less patient movement, and often a more rapid recovery because it essentially uses less drug.

Availability and training in the use of an intraosseous access device is also recommended in facilities that choose to treat children. The placement of an IV in a child requires skill and patience, and can be challenging. The increased incidence of obesity in children poses an added level of difficulty to this. In the event of difficulty in procuring a peripheral vascular access, the most reliable alternative is IO access, especially in an emergency.

Inhalational anesthesia technique

Dentists have been familiar with inhalational anesthesia technique using nitrous oxide since 1844. Nitrous oxide has had a proven wide margin of safety and has few side effects in the pediatric population. It is rapid on induction as well as emergence, and is a potent analgesic. We have known that it causes insignificant cardiovascular and respiratory changes. When added to a second inhalational agent, it promotes anesthesia through second gas effect.

Inhalational techniques are much better tolerated and perceived as less invasive. Typically, a mask is well-accepted by a curious child, especially when an added fruity smell detracts from the unpleasant odor of a plastic mask. In most instances, the anesthetic gas(es) are rapidly delivered and onset of anesthesia is quick. In noncooperative children, crying actually helps, with long deep breathes during crying ensuring that the lungs are filled with the anesthetic agent.

Sevoflurane has become the inhalational agent of choice in most OMS offices. It is a halogenated ether with a fast onset of action and predictable recovery. It has a sweet, slightly pungent fruity odor that enjoys decent patient acceptance. The gas itself does not irritate the airway compared with other options, and induction is characterized by a decreased incidence of breath holding and laryngospasms. It has been proven to be safe to be used with local anesthesia with epinephrine. Standard ASA monitoring including preoperative temperature measurement is recommended while using inhalational agents. If sevoflurane is used for procedures that last more than 30 minutes, it is recommended that continuous invasive temperature monitoring be considered.

In cooperative children, preoxygenation for several minutes before induction is ideal. Sevoflurane can be used as a single inhalational agent or in conjunction with nitrous oxide. Incrementally titrating the gas to effect is ideal. Often, once the patient is past stage II of anesthesia, starting an IV and administering anesthetic drugs through that route is preferred. The gas inhalation is stopped and the patient is maintained on mask or nasal cannula O_2 at that juncture.

In uncooperative children, a single breath technique is effective. The circuit is primed with 8% sevoflurane. Preoxygenation is often not practical in a crying child. The mask is placed with some force, often while the child is seated in the parent's lap. Crying promotes quick inhalation of the concentrated gas and induction is rapid. Upon induction, an IV may be placed, the gases discontinued, and the technique converted to a total IV anesthetic.

It is prudent to consider the placement of an IV in all inhalational anesthetics. This is especially true if the patient is relatively small, obese, or younger, or in any circumstance that the anesthesia provider deems that placement of an IV may be a challenge, especially in the event of an untoward event. That IV may never be used, but serves as a safety net. It is best placed when things are under control and before beginning of the procedure rather than in an emergency or midprocedure.

Halogenated gases are triggers for MH. A focused family and personal history regarding the potential for MH should be discussed with patients and parents before planning an inhalational anesthetic. Facilities that use MH triggering agents are recommended to be prepared for an MH event. This preparation includes storing adequate amounts of dantrolene and practicing how to reconstitute it. Newer dantrolene products have made this process less cumbersome, in addition to reducing the amounts of dantrolene that need to be stored.

Safe Discharge

The concept of safe discharge is often overlooked in our busy practices. Although healthy adults and adolescents may recover rapidly from anesthesia delivered in the OMS office, the pediatric population requires a higher level of care and diligence before discharge. The ASA mandates that recovery be:

> [P]rovided in an area that allows pediatric perioperative care, including the management of postoperative complications and the provision pediatric cardiopulmonary resuscitation, and a provider trained and experienced in pediatric perioperative care, should be made immediately available to evaluate and treat any child in distress. Patient-care facilities (including ambulatory surgical centers) that perform operative procedures for which postoperative intensive care is not anticipated may develop a proactive, clearly delineated plan (ie, a "transfer agreement") to transfer children to an appropriate hospital facility when complications requiring inpatient monitoring/care occur.[8]

Postanesthetic laryngospasms are more common in the pediatric population. Hence, recovery in a lateral position is recommended to avoid secretions irritating chords. State of consciousness, assessment and documentation of vitals, age-appropriate ambulation, pain control, and the absence of postoperative nausea and vomiting is required before discharge. Two responsible adult escorts riding in the same vehicle accompanying a child home is a safe practice after pediatric anesthesia. In the event of narcosis, postdischarge vomiting and aspiration or inadequate postoperative pain control, having a second adult to assist the patient other than the driver of the vehicle simply makes everything safer.

The administration of a reversal agent during the anesthetic would warrant a longer recovery period because many of these agents have a shorter duration of action than the sedative drugs themselves and the risk of resedation is often imminent. A minimum of 1 hour after administration of a reversal agent is recommended to ensure resedation does not occur before discharge. There is no mandated time period for recovery before safe discharge in either adult or pediatric sedation in the OMS office. Most practitioners and institutions adopt a standard discharge criteria documentation such as a modified Aldrete score or a Richmond Agitation-Sedation Scale. Regardless of the method of documenting discharge and recovery, like everything else in pediatric anesthesia, a pinch more of diligence is required to avoid complications in this vulnerable population.

ACCOMMODATING CHILDREN WITH SPECIAL NEEDS

OMSs are seeing an increased presence of children with special needs such as those in the autism spectrum disorders and attention deficit hyperactivity disorders (ADHD) in our offices.

Autism Spectrum Disorders

The Centers for Disease Control and Prevention estimated in 2016 that 1 in 68 children (1 in 42 boys and 1 in 189 girls) have autism in the United States. Children with autism spectrum disorder have varying levels of social communication and interaction as well as other clinical features. This finding suggests that treating these children in the office often requires a level of personalized care especially as it relates to the provision of anesthesia. Some of these patients may be high functional without any psychological or physiologic burden of the condition, and can be essentially treated the same as any other child. The other end of the spectrum might be an extremely uncooperative child with severe behavioral issues who may simply not be an deal candidate for office-based anesthesia. This spectrum of cooperation and the awareness of comorbidities should influence the anesthetic plan.[9]

In general children, with autism spectrum disorder do better in familiar surroundings, predictability, and structure. Keeping consultation visits close to the procedure appointment helps with that. During consultation visits, allow the child to manipulate instruments and materials, such as holding the mask, and consider sending a mask home with the child for them to get familiar with. It helps to engage the child using a mobile app.[10]

For those children with lower-level language abilities, using simple language, speaking clearly, and avoiding abstract language and figures of speech, as well as using visual cues and supports and keeping instructions simple, help tremendously. It helps to take time to know the child's likes, dislikes, favorite activities, negative triggers, and coping techniques, and to involve parents in preoperative decisions. Premedication may be beneficial, especially in those with severe intellectual disability, but be aware that these children have specific likes and dislikes of textures and tastes. Considering mixing in the child's favorite drink in the context of NPO guidelines is a practical tip.[11] Recovering in the presence of parents or a favorite toy for a prolonged period of time is often helpful.

Attention Deficit Hyperactivity Disorder

ADHD is a brain disorder marked by ongoing pattern of inattention and/or hyperactivity–impulsivity that interferes with function or development. It is estimated that world-wide its prevalence is approximately 5% to 7% in children and adolescent (approximately 5% in the United States).[12] Although it is considered a condition of the childhood, about one-half of the time, it persists into adulthood. Males are generally more affected than females. The 3 key behaviors of children with ADHD are:

- Inattention;
- Hyperactivity; and
- Impulsivity.

Although it is normal to have some inattention, unfocused motor activity, and impulsivity in child, in children with ADHD, these are more severe, occur more often, and interfere with or reduce the quality of function socially, at school, or at work. There is no proposed cure for ADHD, but treatment is aimed to reduce symptoms and enhance social function. Modalities of managing ADHD include medications, psychotherapy, education or training, and often a combination of these.

Medications for ADHD basically fall into 2 categories—stimulants and nonstimulants (**Table 5**). The real question for most practitioners is how to manage these medications for office-based anesthesia in these patients. Children with ADHD exhibit significantly less cooperative behavior at the induction of anesthesia as well as increased level of maladaptive behaviors postoperatively, such as an increase in temper tantrums or fidgety behavior. Having said that, there is evidence to suggest that children with and without ADHD undergoing procedural sedation showed that these children were equally sedated with the same total drug dosages.

The literature is also conflicting and scant regarding continuing versus withholding common ADHD medications for general anesthesia. Psychostimulants are thought to increase the risk of hypertension and arrhythmias, decrease the seizure threshold, and blunt the physiologic response to hypotension owing to a depleted catecholamine reserve. However, there are no reports of any cardiovascular instability in patients with chronic amphetamine use undergoing general anesthesia while continuing the amphetamine regimen. Although methylphenidate has a specific contraindication to the concomitant use of a halogenated anesthetic owing to the risk of sudden blood pressure increase, there is not a clear contraindication or evidence-based protocol for continuing or withholding other psychostimulants perioperatively.

When selective serotonin reuptake inhibitors are used as a nonstimulant therapy for ADHD, the anesthesia provider will need to pay close attention bleeding risk owing to possible interaction with platelet aggregation. The anesthesia provider will need to consider the bleeding risk from surgery as well as the severity of the underlying psychiatric problem when considering continuing, switching,

Table 5	
Common medication regimen for attention deficit hyperactivity disorder	
Stimulants	**Nonstimulants**
Amphetamines (Adderall, Vyvanse)	Atomoxetine (Strattera)
Methamphetamine (Desoxyn)	Selective serotonin reuptake inhibitor antidepressants
Methylphenidate (Concerta, Ritalin)	

or discontinuing a selective serotonin reuptake inhibitor in the perioperative period, preferably with a psychiatric consultation.

DRAWING A PERSONAL LINE WITH PEDIATRIC ANESTHESIA

Providing safe anesthetic care in the OMS office is not a trivial task. Recent reports of untoward events and complications that have led to both mortality and morbidity when anesthetics were administered to children outside the operating room setting, especially in dental offices, brings to light the risks and vulnerability of nonanesthesiologists providing anesthesia. Although OMS training programs provide rigorous training and validation of competency in provision of anesthesia outside the operating room, when adverse events occur, all nonanesthesiologists are equally vindicated. Although all OMS training programs in the United States train to the same minimum standards, not all training is the same. Trainees may be exposed to varying quality and quantity of cases during their training.

OMSs who take on the responsibility of offering pediatric anesthesia in their offices must take a hard look at their ability to safely provide it. How young a child are you prepared to anesthetize in the office? Is your office and your staff prepared for anesthetic emergencies in pediatric anesthesia? Is your training and equipment appropriate to perform safe pediatric anesthesia? Do you routinely perform emergency drills with scenarios involving pediatric adverse events? Is performing pediatric anesthesia a risk you need to take on in today's world? That is a personal line that one must draw after reviewing all the factors mentioned (and more) objectively.

SUMMARY

Children are not just small adults. Clear differences in the anatomy and physiology of a child requires additional training, skills, and techniques in performing anesthesia for a child in our offices. This article reviewed the salient differences in the anatomy and physiology of a child as they pertain to the provision of anesthesia in an OMS office. It also reviewed training standards in pediatric anesthesia in OMS training programs and current guidelines for the safe care of these patients in our offices. Common anesthetic techniques were discussed as they pertain to the pediatric population. Further, the management of children

with autism spectrum disorder and ADHD were discussed.

REFERENCES

1. Kliegman, Stanton, St. Geme, et al. Nelson textbook of pediatrics. 20th edition. Elsevier; 2015.
2. Wani TM, Rafiq M, Akhter N, et al. Upper airway in infants-a computed tomography-based analysis. Paediatr Anaesth 2017;27(5):501–5.
3. Wani TM, Bissonnette B, Rafiq Malik M, et al. Age-based analysis of pediatric upper airway dimensions using computed tomography imaging. Pediatr Pulmonol 2016;51(3):267–71.
4. Li CQ, Wang DX, Cheng T, et al. Effects of recent upper respiratory-tract infections on incidence of the perioperative respiratory adverse events in children: a prospective cohort study. Beijing Da Xue Xue Bao Yi Xue Ban 2017;49(5):814–8 [in Chinese].
5. American Dental Association (ADA). Standards for advanced specialty education programs - oral maxillofacial surgery. Available at: http://www.ada.org/media/CODA/Files/oms.pdf. Accessed October 30, 2017.
6. American Association of Oral Maxillofacial Surgeons (AAOMS). Parameters of care 2017 – anesthesia. Available at: https://www.aaoms.org/images/uploads/pdfs/parcare_anesthesia_1.pdf. Accessed November 15, 2017.
7. Practice guidelines for preoperative fasting and the use of pharmacologic agents to reduce the risk of pulmonary aspiration: application to healthy patients undergoing elective procedures -an updated report by the American Society of Anesthesiologists Task Force on preoperative fasting and the use of pharmacologic agents to reduce the risk of pulmonary aspiration. Anesthesiology 2011;114:495–511. Available at: http://anesthesiology.pubs.asahq.org/article.aspx?articleid=1933410. Accessed October 30, 2017.
8. American Society of Anesthesiologists (ASA). Statement on practice recommendations for pediatric anesthesia committee of origin: pediatric anesthesia (Approved by the ASA House of Delegates on October 19, 2011 and reaffirmed on October 26, 2016). Available at: http://www.asahq.org/quality-and-practice-management/standards-guidelines-and-related-resources/statement-on-practice-recommendations-for-pediatric-anesthesia Accessed October 30, 2017.
9. Vlassakova BG, Emmanouil DE. Perioperative considerations in children with autism spectrum disorder. Curr Opin Anaesthesiol 2016;29(3):359–66.
10. Isong IA, Rao SR, Holifield C, et al. Addressing dental fear in children with autism spectrum

disorders: a randomized controlled pilot study using electronic screen media. Clin Pediatr (Phila) 2014; 53(3):230–7.

11. Prakash S, Pai VK, Dhar M, et al. Premedication in an autistic, combative child: challenges and nuances. Saudi J Anaesth 2016;10(3): 339–41.

12. ADHD Institute. Epidemiology of ADHD. Available at: http://www.adhd-institute.com/burden-of-adhd/ epidemiology/. Accessed November 15, 2017.

Oral Surgery Patient Safety Concepts in Anesthesia

Richard C. Robert, DDS, MS*, Chirag M. Patel, DMD, MD

KEYWORDS

- Human error • Crisis resource management • Checklists • Interactive cognitive aids
- In situ simulation • Debriefings

KEY POINTS

- Rather than placing blame on an individual when errors occur, Reason's approach is to modify systems to limit the likelihood of similar errors in the future.
- Crisis resource management provides a foundation for a safe patient treatment environment through effective use of personnel, emergency equipment, medications and supplies, and communication, seeking assistance when necessary.
- An effective office emergency preparedness plan is based on well-designed checklists, use of cognitive aids, and regular in situ emergency simulations.
- Technologic advancements have made it possible to develop interactive cognitive aids that enhance training of team members and provide more rapid access to essential information, during in situ simulations as well as during an actual crisis.
- A debriefing following an in situ simulation exercise is an invaluable teaching tool and provides an opportunity to "troubleshoot" systems, which require revision or updating.

INTRODUCTION

Of all the goals laid out in setting up an oral and maxillofacial surgery (OMS) practice, assuring patient safety is undoubtedly the most important. In reaching that goal, 4 objectives must be considered, 3 of which have been addressed in previous articles of this issue. These include the following:

1. Patient selection and preoperative workup: The patient's history and clinical findings must be carefully reviewed to assure that the patient is a candidate for an office-based anesthetic. The preoperative workup may entail consultation with the patient's primary care physician or other specialists, as well as obtaining appropriate laboratory studies in some cases.

2. Appropriate choice of anesthetic agents and careful delivery: The patient's anesthetic must be catered to his or her age, gender, habitus, and state of medical compromise.

3. Adequate training of the members of the anesthetic team: All members of the surgical and anesthetic team must be well trained and participate in continuing education.

4. An emergency preparedness plan to manage all anticipated untoward events: This article delves into this latter aspect of patient safety.

Managing Human Error

The foundation of a safe patient environment is firmly based on the anticipation of human error

No disclosures regarding financial or commercial interests.
Department of Oral and Maxillofacial Surgery, University of California, San Francisco School of Dentistry, Box 0440, 533 Parnassus Avenue, UB 10, San Francisco, CA 94143, USA
* Corresponding author.
E-mail address: rcr2400@aol.com

Oral Maxillofacial Surg Clin N Am 30 (2018) 183–193
https://doi.org/10.1016/j.coms.2018.01.005
1042-3699/18/© 2018 Elsevier Inc. All rights reserved.

and dealing with it, as well as management of the various resources available for responding to a crisis ("crisis resource management"[1]). Historically, the consequences of human error have been attributed to deficiencies in an individual. He or she is looked upon as being forgetful, inattentive, unintelligent, negligent, or reckless.[2] However, English psychology professor James Reason at the University of Manchester has posited the now widely accepted theory that human errors are more frequently the result of deficiencies in systems as opposed to individuals.[3] He has proposed the "Swiss cheese model," illustrated in **Fig. 1**. In this model, slices of Swiss cheese represent the culture of the operation with the various defenses and safeguards which have been established to prevent losses. However, when holes which have developed in these defenses align, a potential hazard then becomes a loss.

Reason's approach to managing human error is to first create systems that limit the likelihood of an individual error. In surgery, there is considerable stress, such as fatigue due to sleep deprivation, heavy workloads, long commutes, a hierarchal culture, time restraints, and often poor supervision. In this setting, some errors are inevitable and should be anticipated. Thus, systems need to be in place that can detect early on the occurrence of an error and contain its damaging effects before a catastrophic loss takes place.[4]

Crisis resource management

The elements of Crisis Resource Management are directed toward the establishment of systems that satisfy Reason's concepts. As described by Goldhaber-Fiebert and Howard[1] at Stanford Medical Center, there are 11 key points in the implementation of effective crisis resource management. These include the following:

1. Call for help early
2. Designate leadership
3. Establish role clarity
4. Distribute the workload
5. Communicate effectively
6. Anticipate and plan
7. Know the environment
8. Use all available information
9. Allocate attention wisely
10. Mobilize resources
11. Use cognitive aids

In the sections that follow, an emergency preparedness plan for the OMS office based on these key points is described. It was developed by the lead author of this article for the California Association of Oral and Maxillofacial Surgeons (CALAOMS) and the Department of Oral and Maxillofacial Surgery at the University of California at San Francisco. The components of the plan can be found on the CALAOMS Web site and are available to nonmembers as well as CALAOMS members. The Internet address for the folder containing these materials is: https://www.calaoms.org/Robert.

Implementation of the Emergency Preparedness Plan

This plan is implemented through the 3-step process outlined in later discussion. It should be designed and implemented by the surgeon and a staff member designated as the "Emergency Preparedness Coordinator." The coordinator should ideally have experience as an anesthesia assistant and possess good organizational skills. It is his or her responsibility to monitor the various aspects of the office emergency preparedness plan and report to the surgeon on a regular basis (usually monthly) regarding the status of the plan. The process for establishing the plan includes the 3 following components:

1. Development of an office emergency preparedness plan based on well-designed checklists.
2. Incorporation of cognitive aids into the procedures and protocols for the management of anesthetic and medical emergencies.
3. Conducting regularly scheduled emergency simulations based on cognitive aids in the office setting ("in situ") to prepare the office for potential emergencies. These in situ simulations should be augmented with simulation courses offered by professional organizations such as that described in David W. Todd and John J. Schaefer III's article, "The American Association of Oral and Maxillofacial Surgeons (AAOMS) Simulation Program," in this issue.

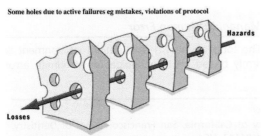

Some holes due to active failures eg mistakes, violations of protocol

Hazards

Losses

Other holes due to latent conditions eg faulty equipment, inexperienced staff

Fig. 1. Reason's Swiss cheese model. (*From* Sarker SK, Vincent C. Errors in surgery. Int J Surg 2005;3(1):77; with permission.)

DEVELOPING WELL-DESIGNED CHECKLISTS

The starting point is deceptively simple lists of resources such as personnel duties, inventory, and maintenance. These lists must be prepared with care to ensure that all critical items are listed. Without these systems in place as a foundation, effective cognitive aids and simulations are not possible.[5] There is ample evidence supporting checklists as indispensable tools in preventing errors in surgery and anesthesia. Surgeon Atul Gawande at the Brigham and Women's Hospital in Boston, Massachusetts has written a *New York Times* Bestseller on their power in managing complexity in medicine.[6] In the next sections, the authors explore some of the checklists that can be used to ensure emergency preparedness of an OMS practice.

Delegation of Duties

The first checklists are used for *delegation of duties for office personnel in a medical emergency crisis*. Office personnel include the surgeon, surgical staff, and the administrative staff. Ideally, the members of the surgical staff are an airway assistant, a second assistant, and a circulator. In the event a medical emergency arises, it should be clear to all personnel what their "new" roles are. The following are 5 important job descriptions that the authors use in their practices that are assigned to the office personnel in the event of a medical or anesthetic emergency:

1. The airway assistant (surgical staff)
   a. Suctioning and airway maintenance
   b. Delivery of positive pressure O_2: This includes connections of face mask and adjusting the O_2 flow
   c. Assist in placement of airway adjuncts such as nasopharyngeal airway, oral pharyngeal airway, laryngeal mask airway, and endotracheal tube
   d. Assist with securing of tubes
   e. Assist with anesthesia machine connections
2. The medication assistant (surgical staff)
   a. Prepare and pass airway adjuncts to surgeon
   b. Retrieve and draw up medications for administration under supervision of surgeon
   c. Delivery of medications under supervision of surgeon
3. The circulator (surgical staff)
   a. Procure the emergency kit or crash cart, airway supplies, defibrillator, and so forth
   b. Prepare and deliver intravenous fluids as directed by surgeon
   c. Chest compressions under direction of surgeon
   d. Defibrillation under supervision of surgeon

4. The scribe (administrative staff)
   a. Obtain vital signs at direction of surgeon
   b. Fill out medical emergency record, including vital signs, events, medications administered, and personnel roles
   c. Complete anesthesia record
   d. When incomplete office records regarding the emergency must be given to the emergency medical technicians (EMTs), they should be marked "Incomplete record—Provided to facilitate patient transfer. Completed record will be faxed to the ER." Then make sure that records are completed STAT and faxed as promised.
5. 911 call assistant (administrative staff)
   a. Fill out 911 form with input from surgeon
   b. Make 911 call
   c. Request that another staff member escort the patient's family member or escort from the waiting room to an unused operatory to advise him or her of the emergency.
   d. Request a staff member to meet the EMTs at the back door
   e. Discharge other patients and escorts from the waiting room

Documenting Drills and Continuing Education Courses

Spreadsheet software such as Microsoft Excel can be used to create a master "Emergency Preparedness Workbook" that consists of worksheets corresponding to the checklists mentioned in later discussion. A yearly emergency preparedness checklist (**Fig. 2**A) is filled out at the beginning of the year to schedule and track drills (familiarity and scenario) and continuing education (CE) courses, such as basic life support and advanced cardiac life support. A scenario drill should be scheduled every quarter with familiarity drills in the 2 previous months (familiarity drills described in later discussion). Two checklists aid in recording staff attendance and proficiency during familiarity drills: one list is for surgical staff (**Fig. 2**C) and another for administrative staff (**Fig. 2**D). An important aspect of these 2 checklists is the concept of staff members' proctoring one other; this ensures adequate completion of the familiarity drills to gain proficiency. Finally, there is a checklist to document staff attendance at scenario drills and CE courses (**Fig. 2**B). In the event of an unfortunate event and litigation, these documents can be invaluable.

Maintenance of Equipment and Associated Supplies

A monthly checklist aids in *maintenance of equipment and associated supplies* (**Fig. 2**E), such as

A

EMERGENCY PREPAREDNESS - YEARLY CHECKLIST			2007		
Date	Assistants	Description	Scheduled For:	Completed	Assistant
01/03/06		1st Familiarity Drill for 1st Quarter 2008 Scenario Drill	Oct. 18, 06		
01/03/06		2nd Familiarity Drill for 1st Quarter 2008 Scenario Drill	Nov. 15, 06		
01/02/07		1st Quarter 2008 Scenario Drill	Jan. 17, 07		

B

EMERGENCY PREPAREDNESS DRILLS AND CE			2007
Date and Time	Drill or CE	Description	In Attendance
Wed., Jan-17, 2007 10:30 AM - 12:30 PM	Drill	Scenario Drill - Respiratory and Cardiovascular I (Vasovar) Emergencies with Dr. Robert	Aurora, Bryan, Sandra, Jason, Alexis, Virginia, Heather
Sat., Feb-24, 2007 8:00 AM	CE	CALAOMS OMSA Course - Set. # AM - 4 PM · Sun. 8 AM - 1 PM	Recertification Jason, Recertification-Alexis, Certification-Virginia
Wed., Apr-18, 2007 6:00 am - 10:30 am	CE	BLS Course - All Staff	Aurora, Bryan, Sandra, Jason, Alexis, Virginia, Heather

C

Familiarity Drills and Proficiency Checklist - Surgical Staff														
Date	Assistant's Name:	Proctor:	Positive Press. O_2	Assist. - Intub. / F.B.Obstr.	Assist. - LMA	Assist. - Cric.	Emerg. O_2 / Suct.	Peak Flow Meter	Proc. Equip. & Drugs	Special Drug Vials	Drug Dilu-tions	Gluco-meter	CPR and Heimlich	Set-up Defib. & Defib.

D

Familiarity Drills and Proficiency Checklist - Administrative Staff													
Date	Administrative Staff Name:	Proctor	911 Call and Form	Handle Escort / Family	Discharge Wtg Room Pt's	Emerg. O_2 / Suct.	Set-up Defib & Defib.	Vital Signs - Machine	Vital Signs - Manual	Medical Emerg. Form	Proc. Equip.	CPR and Heimlich

E

EMERGENCY PREPAREDNESS - MONTHLY CHECKLIST													Dec-2007
DATE	T O C H E C K	ASSISTANT	WALL CLOCKS (WKLY)	MONITOR CLOCKS (WKLY)	OPERATORY INVENTORY (WEEKLY)			ANESTH. BAGS	FLASHLIGHTS (WEEKLY)		PORT. O_2	T O C H E C K	AED	COMMENTS
					ROOM 2	ROOM 4	AIRWAYK IT	WEEKLY	PLGD	WRKG	WKLY		MONTHLY	
Mon., Dec-03, 2007														
Tue., Dec-04, 2007													✓	

F

EMERGENCY MEDICATIONS AND SUPPLIES LOG						
Date Received	Emerg,	Drug/Concentration	Size of Vial	Expiration Date	Month to Re-Order	Date Ordered
Filter					Filter	Filter
7/20/06	ACS-Angina	Nitroglycerin .4 mg tablet	25 tb btl	2008, Mar.	2008, Feb. ▼	
3/10/07	ACS-Angina	Nitroglycerin spray .4 mg/dose	12 Gm btl	2008, Jun.	2008, Apr.	
7/5/07	ACS-Myocardial Infarction	Aspirin 325 mg (chewable tabs)	100tb/btl	2008, Dec.	2008, Oct.	

Fig. 2. Actual individual spreadsheets from the Emergency Preparedness Workbook as discussed in the text (*A–F*). The spreadsheets are available from the CALAOMS website.

wall clocks, monitor clocks, operatory equipment, airway adjuncts and supplies, flashlights, portable oxygen (**Fig. 3**), backup suction, and automated external defibrillator (AED). Most items should be checked on a weekly basis except the AEDs, which only need to be checked on a monthly basis.

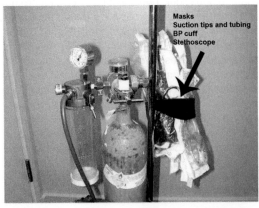

Fig. 3. Portable oxygen tank with relevant emergency equipment.

Masks
Suction tips and tubing
BP cuff
Stethoscope

Organization of Emergency Drugs and Equipment

An *Emergency Drugs and Supplies* checklist (**Fig. 2**F) helps to organize and ensure these items are ordered before the expiration date. Drugs are listed by type of medical emergency (sorted alphabetically), such as allergic reaction, angina, bronchospasm/asthma, cardiac dysrhythmias, etc. This list also includes all nonmedication items that have expiration dates, such as pads for the defibrillator, batteries for atomic clocks, endotracheal tubes and supraglottic airways. Placing a "Z" before the name of each of these latter items AND the emergency for which they are used will place them at the bottom of the list. The expiration date is listed alongside the month to reorder, which is 2 months earlier to allow for ordering and receiving the item before expiration. The Microsoft Excel Filter function can be used to filter by current month and year to enable timely reordering[7] (**Fig. 4**).

Ordering and Inventory

A master office supplies inventory list is also maintained in the form of a Microsoft Excel

A

Emerg.	EMERGENCY DRUG/Conc. or SUPPLY	Size of Vial	Expiration Date	Month to Re-Order	Date Ordered	Date Received
Dysr. - Tachy - NAR. - REG. (SVT)	Adenosine 6 mg/2 mL	2 mL SDV	2017, Dec.	2017, Oct.		6
Z-Supplies	ADULT QUICKTACH (emergency cricithrotomy device)		2/1/21	12/1/20		6
Z-Supplies	Aerobic/Anaerobic Culturette Collection Swab	50/box	5/31/18	3/31/18		6
Asthma / Bronchospasm	Albuterol Inhaler 90 mcgm/puff	17 gm spry. can	2017, Nov.	2017, Sep.		15
Dysr. - Tachy - VF / VT (pulseless)	Amiodarone 150 mg / 3 mL	3 mL SDV	2017, Oct.	2017, Aug.		17
Dysr. - Tachy - WIDE - V.T.	Amiodarone 150 mg / 3 mL	3 mL SDV	2017, Oct.	2017, Aug.		17
Syncope	Ammonia Inhalant 3 mL/vial	.33 mL caps.	2019, Dec.	2019, Oct.		17
Z-Supplies	Anaerobe System Culture Test Packet w/ swab	Unit Box	6/19/17	4/19/17		17
ACS-Myocardial Infarction	Aspirin 325 mg (chewable tabs)	100tb/btl	2017, Dec.	2017, Oct.		15
Dysr. - Asyst. / PEA	Atropine .4 mg/mL	20 mL MDV	2018, Feb.	2017, Dec.		16
Dysr. - Bradycardia (Sympt.)	Atropine .4 mg/mL	20 mL MDV	2018, Feb.	2017, Dec.		10/3/16
Emesis and Aspiration	Bacteriostatic Sodium Chloride .9%	30 mL MDV	2018, Aug.	2018, Jun.		1/18/17
Z-Supplies	Battery-AED - Power Stick 4+	1 ea	2018, Oct.	2018, Aug.		7/16/13
Z-Supplies	Battery-Atomic Clock- Size AA (In-use change 18 mo)	1 pkg of 36	2023, Dec.	2023, Oct.		2/5/14
Z-Supplies	Battery-Laryngoscope - Size C	1 pkg of 4	2023, Dec.	2023, Oct.		1/21/09
Allergic Reaction	Benadryl 50 mg/cc	1 mL MDV	2018, Mar.	2018, Jan.		5/19/16
Hiccups	Chlorpromazine 25 mg/cc	1 mL SDV	2017, Oct.	2017, Aug.		11/9/15
Z-Supplies	D5W w/ Dextrose (procainamide, magnesium sulfate: kit)	250 mL	9/1/17	7/1/17		1/18/17
Allergic Reaction	Decadron 4 mg/cc	30 mL MDV	2018, Feb.	2017, Dec.		3/1/16
Insulin Shock	Dextrose Inj. 50% .5 g/mL	50 mL SDV	3/1/18	1/1/18		4/5/17
Seizure	Diazepam 5 mg/mL	10 mL MDV	2017, Sep.	2017, Jul.		2/10/16
Z-Supplies	Dieckmann Intraosseous Infusion Needle	16 G/3 cm	10/19/21	8/19/21		3/28/17
Dysr. - Tachy - NAR. - IRREG.	Diltiazem 25 mg/5 mL (Fridge)	5 mL SDV	2019, Jan.	2018, Nov.		4/4/17

B

Emerg.	EMERGENCY DRUG/Conc. or SUPPLY	Size of Vial	Expiration Date	Month to Re-Order	Date Ordered	Date Received
Dysr. - Tachy - VF / VT (pulseless)	Amiodarone 150 mg / 3 mL	3 mL SDV	2017, Oct.	2017, Aug.		1/18/17
Dysr. - Tachy - WIDE - V.T.	Amiodarone 150 mg / 3 mL	3 mL SDV	2017, Oct.	2017, Aug.		1/18/17
Hiccups	Chlorpromazine 25 mg/cc	1 mL SDV	2017, Oct.	2017, Aug.		11/9/15

Fig. 4. Screenshots from Microsoft Excel showing the Filter function in action. (*A*) Filter function is activated by clicking on the dropdown arrow in the Month to Re-Order cell. This month is selected. (*B*) The drugs due for ordering this month are populated and can be easily ordered.

spreadsheet.[8] Orders are placed by faxing an order form developed in an Excel spreadsheet from the items in the master office inventory list. Once the order has been received, the items should be checked off on the order form to assure that the appropriate items have been received (**Fig. 5**). An important aspect of this process is accountability. The person who performs the task records his or her initials and the date. The purpose of this is to prevent serious errors, such as using the wrong drug. For example, if D50W is received and used

in error when in fact D5W was ordered, the consequences can be devastating.

INCORPORATION OF COGNITIVE AIDS INTO OFFICE PROCEDURES AND PROTOCOLS FOR THE MANAGEMENT OF ANESTHETIC AND MEDICAL EMERGENCIES

As discussed earlier, stress predisposes to errors because of cognitive lapses, especially in an environment of heightened stress such as that

Vendor:

Company Name: Southern Anesthesia & Surgical
Address: 204 Palmetto Park Blvd.
City, State & Zip: Lexington, SC 29072
Phone and Fax: (800) 624-5926   (800) 344-1237

Qty	Units	Product Nuumber	Description	
2	BOX	5110	Alcohol Prep Sterile Large	200 per
3	Bx	BP1215	Blade No. 15 - Stainless Steel	- Bard
2	PKG	2181	Double Stick Disc	3M
1	Box	4311L	Medex Large body Stopcock 3 way with male luer slip	
40	BTL	66758001801	Midazolam 1 mg - mL - 10 mL MDV	
6	BOX	32138	Syringe - 3 cc with 21g X 1 1 - 2 in. - Terumo - 100 - box	
1	box	08TU05L101	Syringe - 5 cc syringe only - 100 - box - Terumo	
1	box	10L	Syringe-10 cc syringe only - 100 - box - Terumo Luer Lock	
6	BOX	06TU032138	Syringes - 3 cc Terumo brand with needle 21x1 1 - 2 in. -	
10	BTL	42023011310	Ketalar 10 mg/mL 20 mL MDV	

Fig. 5. Checklist used for confirming receipt of correct items. Please note that the person who performs this task signs and dates the document. This ensures accountability in case an error is made.

which accompanies an anesthetic or medical emergency. Memory or cognitive lapses can thus lead to anesthetic catastrophes, with fatal consequences. In the field of aviation, such stress-induced errors have been countered by incorporation of cognitive aids. When the first B-17 bomber crashed and burned on its maiden flight because of failure by the pilot to flip a switch, a preflight checklist was developed.[6] When commercial aviation fatalities began to increase to catastrophic levels in the 1960s, the industry again turned to cognitive aids as a major thrust in their crusade for airline safety. Between 1965 and 2010, fatalities dropped from 5564 to 0.011 fatalities per hundred flight hours. It was found that the cognitive aids that were most effective in achieving this dramatic improvement were simple and "user friendly."[4]

Incorporation of cognitive aids into office procedures and protocols for the management of anesthetic and medical emergencies can significantly improve patient outcomes. Four vital elements for implementing cognitive aids, such as emergency manuals, are the following: create (content and design), familiarize (training), use (access and roles), and integrate (culture).[1] Unfortunately, the greatest hindrance to effective use of cognitive aids is the classic mentality that "doctors know everything" and do not need crutches such as cognitive aids.

An intriguing aspect of the development of cognitive aids is the potential for the use of technology to make the aids more effective. Office automation can empower organizational concepts in the establishment of emergency response systems. Interactive aids made possible by office automation can enable more rapid retrieval of information and guidance in the application of appropriate interventions. What follows is a brief description of cognitive aids incorporated into the authors' practices.

Intuitive System for Organization of Drugs and Equipment

In keeping with a simple and "user-friendly" approach found to be so effective in the aviation industry, the organization of drugs in the crash cart relies on a simple alphabetical arrangement that is logical and intuitive. Drugs are arranged in alphabetical order *of the emergency* for which they are used (**Fig. 6**A). When more than one drug is required for treatment of an emergency, all drugs required for that emergency are stored together. For example, epinephrine, diphenhydramine, ranitidine, and dexamethasone are stored

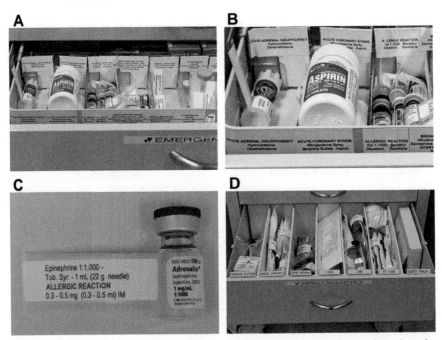

Fig. 6. Cognitive aids useful in an OMS practice. (*A*) Alphabetical arrangement of drugs based on the emergency for which they are used. (*B*) When multiple drugs are required, they are all stored together in a single bin. (*C*) Vial of epinephrine with attached label containing the essential information to enable error-free delivery of the drug for treatment of an allergic reaction. (*D*) Arrangement of airway adjuncts in the order they would be used in an emergency situation based on the difficult airway algorithm.

together in a single compartment for management of allergic reactions (**Fig. 6**B).

It is beyond the scope of this article to review every emergency drug that should be included in an OMS crash cart. However, a recent advancement involving the introduction of the drug sugammadex[9] warrants a brief discussion. Sugammadex is a reversal agent for non-depolarizing muscle relaxants such as rocuronium. Rocuronium can be used as a replacement for succinylcholine for the treatment of laryngospasm. It is inexpensive and does not have the potential risk of inducing malignant hyperthermia, the treatment of which requires storage of dantrolene. Although the new reversal agent sugammadex is somewhat expensive, it can be stocked in the OMS office for approximately $80 to $90 per year.

Effective Utilization of Labeling Enabled by Office Automation

Appropriate drug dosing is very important because a mistake can lead to a patient fatality. Unfortunately, drug retrieval, dosage, and administration are adversely affected by stress in an emergency situation. To overcome this, emergency drug vials are labeled with all information required for administration (**Fig. 6**C). Well-designed labels have been found to enhance safety of medication administration in anesthesia practice.[10] Consequently, labels prepared with office automation have been designed to prevent errors. Information on the labels includes the following:

1. Emergency for which the drug is used
2. Dose in milligrams and milliliters
3. Route of administration
4. Size and type of syringe used for administration

Airway equipment is also organized in an intuitive manner, that is, in the order of the difficult airway algorithm that would be used in an emergency (**Fig. 6**D). Organization and labeling of these items in this way also enables rapid visual inventory. Rather than having to pore over long hardcopy lists of items, the staff can assess at a glance the items being inventoried. The visual inventory concept also enhances staff training. Because checking of airway adjuncts and supplies is a part of the weekly checklist, each anesthesia assistant is familiarized with the organization of the system, the location of the items, and their appearance on a rotating basis.

Interactive Emergency Algorithm PDF

As stated above, stress can impair memory and cognition, which can result in an inability of team members to respond appropriately in a crisis. Several studies have found that these lapses in memory can be countered by well-designed cognitive aids.[1,11,12] Interestingly, not all of the studies in which cognitive aids have been used found them to be of significant benefit. The reasons appeared to be largely attitudinal and cultural. In several cases, the team-leader doctors thought that the use of a cognitive aid was a reflection of a lack of confidence or knowledge. In other cases, there was little participation of the team leaders in the development of the aids, and they were distributed to team members with little if any explanation of how they were to be used.[13] In addition, when training and use of the cognitive aids during simulations were discontinued after initial success, the positive effect was not sustained.[14] In an attempt to overcome some of these potential shortcomings, an interactive Emergency Algorithm PDF was developed. Its use is illustrated in **Fig. 7** and discussed later.

In many current OMS offices, the patient's radiograph is displayed on a computer monitor during the surgical procedure (see **Fig. 7**A). The interactive Emergency Algorithm PDF is opened but hidden behind the radiograph on the monitor screen. In the event of an emergency, with a click of the mouse an anesthesia assistant can bring the Table of Contents of the Emergency Algorithm PDF to the front of the display (see **Fig. 7**B). The algorithms are listed alphabetically by emergency, which match the filing and storage of the emergency drugs in the crash cart, as well as the drug vial labels discussed earlier. The algorithms are accessed by clicking on the name of the emergency, which is a hyperlink leading to the algorithm page (see **Fig. 7**C). If the need for a special procedure is encountered during an algorithm, a hyperlink (signified by a green highlight) can be activated with a mouse click to navigate to the specific special procedure (see **Fig. 7**D).

Each algorithm is accompanied by a page with pathophysiology (not illustrated here) that can be used during training and simulations to review the pertinent details of the specific emergency and the rationale for its treatment. The special procedures alluded to earlier are included in an appendix, which is located at the end of the document to enable rapid access to these procedures.

Regularly Scheduled In Situ Simulations Based on Cognitive Aids

Both lecture and hands-on courses on medical simulation are now available through various medical, dental, and surgical associations, including the American Association of Oral and Maxillofacial

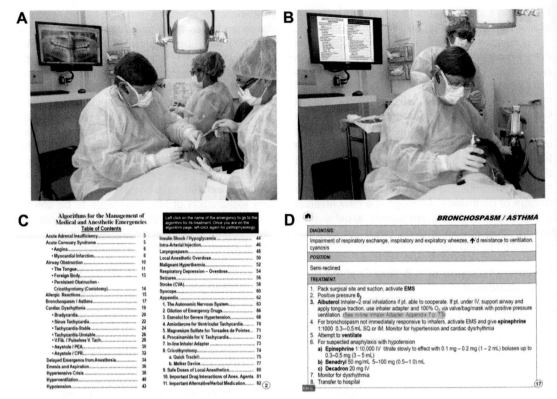

Fig. 7. (*A*) Provider performing surgery with panoramic radiograph on the screen. (*B*) In an emergency situation, the interactive emergency algorithm (IEA) PDF can be retrieved with ease as seen on the screen. (*C*) Contents of the IEA PDF that are hyperlinked to detailed algorithms for quick and easy access. (*D*) Details of the bronchospasm/asthma algorithm with hyperlink to an appendix on Inhaler Adapter.

Surgeons as covered in David W. Todd and John J. Schaefer III's article, "The American Association of Oral and Maxillofacial Surgeons (AAOMS) Simulation Program," in this issue. This coursework should be complemented by regularly scheduled in situ simulations in the same office setting and with the same team members with which the surgeon performs his or her surgical procedures.[15,16]

Familiarity drills

During these drills, the members of the team familiarize themselves with drugs, equipment, and supplies and simulate the individual tasks that will be required in the actual management of emergencies. The development of expertise in the performance of these core skills by individual team members is essential to the success of full simulations. Inadequate training and practice of these skills can lead to a failed response and a fatal outcome in a real emergency crisis.[17] The team members are guided through their familiarity drills with an interactive Emergency Skill Tutorial PDF as cognitive aids (**Fig. 8**A). This aid is automated in a

manner similar to that used for the Automated Medical Emergency Algorithm PDF described earlier.

The familiarity drills are conducted by staff during "downtime," for example, when the surgeon is at a hospital or dental society meeting, CE course, or so forth. Checklists in the "Emergency Preparedness Workbook" as described previously are maintained to document these drills. In addition to checklists for surgical assistants, there are also checklists for the duties of administrative personnel during an emergency. Accountability is essential; the drills should be monitored by another assistant and the monitor noted on the checklist. Personnel should be cross-trained such that all critical team positions are competently staffed in the event of a real emergency.[18]

Team simulations (scenario drills)

During these simulations, the entire treatment team, including administrative personnel, is present, and their duties are simulated along with those of the surgical team (**Fig. 8**B). A fictitious

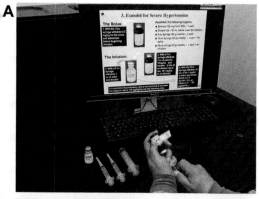

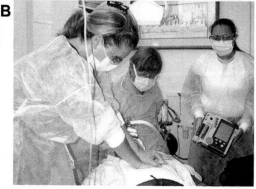

Fig. 8. In situ simulations. (*A*) A familiarity drill in progress involving dilution of Esmolol with the interactive tutorial PDF on the screen. (*B*) A scenario drill in progress with the surgeon controlling the airway and the surgical staff carrying out various tasks.

emergency scenario is outlined by the team leader, and all members of the team participate in the management of the emergency using the skills that they have acquired during their familiarity drills. The "reader"[19] literally reads off the steps in the algorithm from the Automated Emergency Algorithm PDF (see **Fig. 7**) to guide the team through the steps in the algorithm. Accurate, contemporaneous recording of all events, interventions, doses, and so forth is enabled by the Medical Emergency Record (**Fig. 9**) and 911 Call Record (included on the CALAOMS Web site but not illustrated here). Note that little writing is required on the Medical Emergency Record. All of the emergencies, elements of the diagnosis, drugs, and interventions have already been printed on the form. Consequently, all that must be written are drug dosages and numbers signifying the timing of events.

Every attempt should be made by the team members to "suspend disbelief" during conduction of the team simulation.[20] All team members should act and think as if the emergency were actually taking place. These simulations are "rehearsals," so that in the event that an emergency actually occurs, the members of the office staff can perform as a precision emergency response team, just as they did in their rehearsals. Closed loop communication is used throughout, providing verification that essential steps have been followed correctly. As was pointed out earlier, hierarchal posturing has been shown to undermine the effectiveness of cognitive aids and simulations in general. Similarly, it can detract from the effectiveness of simulations when the team leader does not feel that he or she needs "cheat sheets" or input from lesser-trained team members.[21] Whenever possible, a video recording should be made for utilization during debriefings and training of new office personnel.[22] With the advent of "smart phones," making video recordings has been made quite simple.

Debriefing

Immediately following the team simulations, the simulation session should be reviewed with the team members, ideally using the video recording of the simulation.[23] During the debriefing, all members of the team should avoid placing blame and finding fault. Rather they should learn from errors and shortcomings encountered during the simulations.[24] The lessons learned should be recorded and appropriate system changes made to improve protocols as needed. It should be remembered that this is a dynamic process[25] and that improvements in current systems may take place on a regular basis as these simulations are conducted.

SUMMARY

An effective office emergency preparedness plan for the OMS office can be developed through the use of well-designed checklists, cognitive aids, and regularly scheduled in situ simulations with debriefings. In order to achieve this goal, the hierarchal culture of medicine and dentistry must be overcome, and an inclusive team concept must be embraced by all members of the staff. Technologic advancements in office automation now make it possible to create interactive cognitive aids. These aids enhance office emergency training and provide a means for more rapid retrieval of essential information and guidance during both simulations and a real crisis. Regularly scheduled familiarity drills and in situ scenario-based simulations help assure effective emergency response in an actual anesthetic or medical crisis. Debriefings, ideally accompanied by video recordings of simulations, enhance learning and

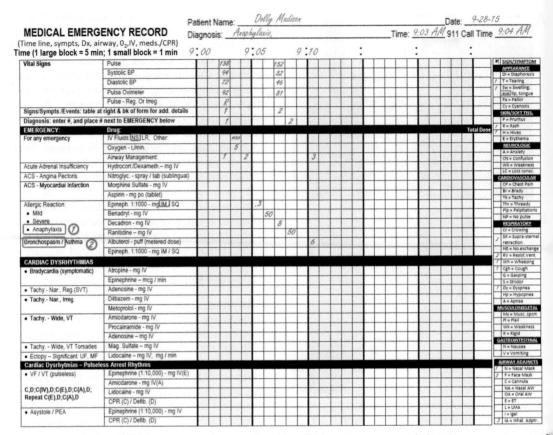

Fig. 9. An example of the front page of a completed medical emergency record showing management of anaphylaxis and bronchospasm.

enable "troubleshooting" of emergency preparedness systems.

REFERENCES

1. Goldhaber-Fiebert SN, Howard SK. Implementing emergency manuals: can cognitive aids help translate best practices for patient care during acute events? Anesth Analg 2013;117(5):1149–61.

2. Reason J. Human error: models and management. BMJ 2000;320(7237):768–70.

3. Reason J. Beyond the organisational accident: the need for "error wisdom" on the frontline. Qual Saf Health Care 2004;13(Suppl 2):ii28–33.

4. Low D, Walker I, Heitmiller ES, et al. Implementing checklists in the operating room. Paediatr Anaesth 2012;22(10):1025–31.

5. Hales B, Terblanche M, Fowler R, et al. Development of medical checklists for improved quality of patient care. Int J Qual Health Care 2008;20(1):22–30.

6. Gawande A. The checklist manifesto: how to get things right. 1st edition. New York: Metropolitan Books; 2010. p. 209, x.

7. Meyer DA, Avery LM. Excel as a qualitative data analysis tool. Field Meth 2009;21(1):91–112.

8. Winters BD, Gurses AP, Lehmann H, et al. Clinical review: checklists - translating evidence into practice. Crit Care 2009;13(6):210.

9. Meistelman C, Donati F. Do we really need sugammadex as an antagonist of muscle relaxants in anesthesia? Curr Opin Anaesthesiol 2016;29(4):462–7.

10. Merry AF, Shipp DH, Lowinger JS. The contribution of labelling to safe medication administration in anaesthetic practice. Best Pract Res Clin Anaesthesiol 2011;25(2):145–59.

11. Gaba DM. Perioperative cognitive aids in anesthesia: what, who, how, and why bother? Anesth Analg 2013;117(5):1033–6.

12. Harrison TK, Manser T, Howard SK, et al. Use of cognitive aids in a simulated anesthetic crisis. Anesth Analg 2006;103(3):551–6.

13. Marshall S. The use of cognitive aids during emergencies in anesthesia: a review of the literature. Anesth Analg 2013;117(5):1162–71.

14. Miller D, Crandall C, Washington C 3rd, et al. Improving teamwork and communication in trauma care through in situ simulations. Acad Emerg Med 2012;19(5):608–12.

15. Miller KK, Riley W, Davis S, et al. In situ simulation: a method of experiential learning to promote safety

and team behavior. J Perinat Neonatal Nurs 2008;
22(2):105–13.

16. Lighthall GK, Poon T, Harrison TK. Using in situ
simulation to improve in-hospital cardiopulmonary
resuscitation. Jt Comm J Qual Patient Saf 2010;
36(5):209–16.

17. Haller G, Laroche T, Clergue F. Morbidity in anaesthesia: today and tomorrow. Best Pract Res Clin
Anaesthesiol 2011;25(2):123–32.

18. DeVita MA, Schaefer J, Lutz J, et al. Improving medical emergency team (MET) performance using a
novel curriculum and a computerized human patient
simulator. Qual Saf Health Care 2005;14(5):326–31.

19. Burden AR, Carr ZJ, Staman GW, et al. Does every
code need a "reader?" Improvement of rare event
management with a cognitive aid "reader" during a
simulated emergency: a pilot study. Simul Healthc
2012;7(1):1–9.

20. Gaba DM. The future vision of simulation in health
care. Qual Saf Health Care 2004;13(Suppl 1):i2–10.

21. Conley DM, Singer SJ, Edmondson L, et al. Effective
surgical safety checklist implementation. J Am Coll
Surg 2011;212(5):873–9.

22. Scherer LA, Chang MC, Meredith JW, et al. Video-
tape review leads to rapid and sustained learning.
Am J Surg 2003;185(6):516–20.

23. Hamilton NA, Kieninger AN, Woodhouse J, et al.
Video review using a reliable evaluation metric
improves team function in high-fidelity simulated
trauma resuscitation. J Surg Educ 2012;69(3):
428–31.

24. Rosen MA, Hunt EA, Pronovost PJ, et al. In situ simulation in continuing education for the health care professions: a systematic review. J Contin Educ Health
Prof 2012;32(4):243–54.

25. Emanuel L, Berwick D, Conway J, et al. What exactly
is patient safety? In: Henriksen K, et al, editors.
Advances in patient safety: new directions and alternative approaches. Rockville (MD): Vol. 1: Assessment; 2008.

The American Association of Oral and Maxillofacial Surgeons Simulation Program

David W. Todd, DMD, MD[a], John J. Schaefer III, MD[b],*

KEYWORDS

- Simulation training • Patient safety • Airway management • Team training • Mastery-based practice
- Cooperative learning

KEY POINTS

- Patient safety in office-based dental anesthesia needs to be improved so that the public, regulators, and patients can be assured that practitioners are competent.
- Simulation training offers doctors the ability to deliberately practice airway management, prepare for adverse events, and learn sedation techniques.
- Past simulation courses in dental anesthesia have not been successful because of excess cost and lack of standardization, objective grading criteria, and a database collection mechanism to support reporting across multiple sites.
- The American Association of Oral and Maxillofacial Surgeons (AAOMS) simulation program will be regionally available and offer a practical cost structure, objective grading criteria, and automatic data collection to support reporting, validation research, and quality assurance.
- The AAOMS simulation program will consist of 3 parts: a course focused primarily on basic emergency airway management, a course on preparation for office-based team crisis management, and a course on intravenous sedation.

INTRODUCTION

Simulation training in anesthesia has been used over the past decade in an attempt to improve patient safety and better prepare clinicians to handle a variety of adverse events that can occur in an anesthetic case. Simulation offers deliberate practice of rare, potentially life-threatening events, evaluation of knowledge and skills, and development of teamwork and communication without the threat of harming real patients. At present, simulation training has developed to the point that it may be possible to assess a clinician's competency to perform treatment. This article focuses on the efforts of the American Association of Oral and Maxillofacial Surgeons (AAOMS) to improve anesthesia safety for oral and maxillofacial surgeons (OMSs) using simulation. This article describes the challenges to improving patient safety in office-based dental anesthesia, the history of the AAOMS simulation program, the current status of the program, and the future of the program as it relates to office-based anesthesia.

Disclosure Statement: Dr Schaefer receives royalties through MUSC for a obstetrical simulation patent licensed by MUSC to Laerdal Medical. Dr Schaefer is currently receiving grant support from a US Department of Defense healthcare obstetrical simulation project. Dr Schaefer received grant support to MUSC from AAOMS for this project.

[a] Private Practice, 120 Southwestern Drive, Lakewood, NY 14750, USA; [b] Department of Anesthesia and Perioperative Medicine, Medical University of South Carolina, 167 Ashley Avenue, Suite 301, MSC 912, Charleston, SC 29425-9120, USA
* Corresponding author.
E-mail address: jjs3md@gmail.com

THE CHALLENGE OF PATIENT SAFETY

In recent years, the safety of office-based anesthesia in the dental field has been called into question. Pediatric dentists, general dentists, OMSs, and dental anesthesiologists have had in-office deaths related to anesthesia administration. Although every death related to health care treatment is a tragedy for all involved, there is a difference in regulator, media, law makers, and general public perception of risk, rates of occurrence, and outcomes when a death occurs in an office versus hospital setting. Adverse events in hospitals are unlikely to be sensationalized in headlines the way that office-based events are, and true rates of adverse events in office settings are more difficult to determine given the emotional toll they take on involved parties. Regardless of the actual rate of occurrence of adverse events, office-based dental anesthesia needs to improve, and patient safety needs to be addressed and enhanced.

It is clear that OMS and all other fields of dentistry need to dedicate themselves to minimizing risk and improving outcomes of office-based anesthesia. As might be expected, a variety of adverse events can occur when performing office-based anesthesia, and severe morbidity and mortality outcomes often occur when the requirement for timely emergency airway management is not adequately provided. There are many challenges to improving patient safety in dentistry, one of which is that in an office environment, there are not many emergency resources readily available. Crisis team training (CTT) for all of the most common emergencies as well as familiarity with emergency drugs and equipment necessary for treatment must be performed frequently enough to maintain staff competency. The AAOMS Office Anesthesia Evaluation (OAE) program was developed more than 20 years ago and standardizes approaches for the facility, team members, emergency drugs, and emergency equipment for office anesthesia. The program has been updated regularly since its inception and provides a good foundation for patient safety; however, it cannot truly measure the competency of a clinician or team in an objective, standardized way. The AAOMS hopes to establish an anesthesia registry in the near future to study true occurrence rates for a variety of outcomes to understand trends and make educated plans for improvement. For most procedures an OMS performs, the procedural risk is low and not a determinant in the location of the procedure, office or hospital. But the first step to improving patient safety begins with proper patient selection: the responsible office anesthesia team must be able to exclude patients who are not good candidates for office-based surgery because of medical history or the results from a physical or airway examination. The competent application of patient safety principles applied to the delivery of anesthetic and sedation practices, concomitant with vigilant monitoring and patient recovery practices, can prevent or mitigate potential patient safety risks. Critical incidents can and will occur despite best practice patient safety care. Therefore, practices must maintain emergency equipment and medications, individual knowledge, and competency in the application of office-based, crisis team practices. AAOMS is committed to improving patient safety through the AAOMS OAE program, coupled with regional training opportunities for meaningful continuing education (CE). The trainings will apply simulation best practice training principles like those in use for commercial aviation simulated emergencies training.

One of the challenges to improving patient safety is the wide variety of practitioners performing office-based anesthesia in the dental field, including general dentists, pediatric dentists, OMSs, dental anesthesiologists, and other specialists. These groups have great variability in training and practitioner experience, and the states in which they practice have different anesthesia regulations and unique laws with contrasting definitions, permitting processes, and training requirements. Many states are just now defining increased requirements for treating pediatric patients under moderate sedation or general anesthetic, while most still allow treatment of pediatric patients if practitioners can satisfy the requirements for a general anesthetic permit regardless of whether the practitioner has experience with pediatric patients. The already steep challenge in standardizing patient safety is exacerbated by political division within dentistry. Some "general dentists" in the American Dental Association (ADA) believe that actions to further regulate and improve patient safety infringe on their right to practice. The goal and focus should be on patient safety, and optimizing patient safety will entail the collaboration of all dentists who provide dental anesthesia.

Concepts to improve patient safety are listed in **Box 1**, which reveals that most of these concepts can be addressed with simulation. **Box 2** describes what effective simulation can achieve.[1] Whether or not simulation is effective depends on the question asked. Simulation is a broad term that can include task trainers, human patient simulation, mannequin-based simulation, or virtual reality. It also depends on how it is structured, used, and measured.[2–6] Generally, in a variety of applications, skill transfers have been well documented. Educational outcomes (knowledge transfer) for some applications are also well

Box 1
Concepts to improve patient safety

- Patient care teams must be prepared to handle rare but potentially life-threatening emergencies.
- The team must be effective with communication, emergency algorithms, and emergency equipment.
- Emergency drills must be regular and as realistic as possible.
- Safety/equipment checklists and written protocols must be performed daily.
- BMV training and supraglottic airway training must take place routinely to maintain competence.
- Patient selection criteria must be followed for pediatric and adult patients.
- Patient monitoring must be understood (especially end-tidal CO_2 and pulse oximetry) by all care team members.

documented and for simulation are at least equal to or slightly better than nonsimulation activities. Less well-proved is transfer of nontechnical skills, such as leadership and communication skills. Also

Box 2
What simulation offers

- Provides active and experiential learning
- Assesses clinician and team competency
- Provides familiarization with emergency equipment and medications to practice rare adverse events
- Gives practitioners the opportunity to
  - Increase patient safety awareness and help to create a culture of safety in the local environment
  - Organize, optimize, and test office emergency operations
  - Make a diagnosis/treatment—think and practice thinking
  - Learn to use checklists and cognitive aids during an emergency
  - Learn and use principles of crew resource management
  - Share best practices
  - Perform deliberate practice for key skills (airway)
  - If data driven, can create national benchmarks from which to compare individual and team readiness to drive meaningful public patient safety standards

lacking are clinical outcomes after simulation training for patient populations in health care organizations, although some examples exist.[7,8] Generalizations in clinical care for simulation may be also hard to prove in terms of translation of successful rehearsal for a critical event in simulation to successful management in routine care or if success in one simulated scenario transfers to another. Although simulation in health care is still in many cases not fully developed, it is widely accepted in use for other high-risk, high-cost industries, such as commercial aviation, shipping, military, and aerospace. In many cases, maintaining certification through simulation or exercise is tied to federal law. In these uses, valid critical fidelity, standardization, and the ability to collect and report performance metric data are critical. One major problem for proving efficacy for a program like the AAOMS simulation course is that major morbidity and mortality are rare events, and therefore documenting a reduction in such events will take a substantial number of cases to have an impact on the rate. Realistically, the next steps that can be taken quickly include (1) validation of the simulation clinical fidelity for its specific use, (2) confirmation of assessment interator reliability, (3) validation of educational outcomes, (4) validation of standardized generalizability across multiple sites, and (5) determination of predictive validity of basic airway management skills assessment and training. It is a priority for AAOMS to assess these parameters with the new simulation CE program.

PAST SIMULATION COURSES

In 2008, the AAOMS Committee on Anesthesia (CAN) in conjunction with dental anesthesiologist colleagues, notably Drs James Phero and Morton Rosenberg, developed a simulation program (using SimMan simulators [Laerdal Medical, Norway]), which was held at the AAOMS national meeting. The simulation program allowed AAOMS members to understand the potential for simulation through simulation mannequins, simulation operators, and facilitators. The program was a 4-hour course in which a group of participants, mostly OMSs and some OMS office teams, participated at various stations. In groups, participants were exposed to a variety of scenarios of possible medical emergencies, and knowledge and treatment were evaluated. In addition to 2 simulation stations, an "airway station" was created in which RespiTrainers (Ingmar Medical, Pittsburgh, Pennsylvania) were used to demonstrate airway manipulations, video laryngoscopes were available for demonstration, intraosseous access was demonstrated, and cardiopulmonary resuscitation (CPR) was demonstrated with feedback device mannequins. The SimMan course was offered at AAOMS national meetings and held in ballrooms laid out for the course. Additionally, the American Dental Society of Anesthesiology has been conducting simulation courses with similar programs and goals for pediatric and adult moderate sedation and deep sedation/general anesthesia.

The goals of the first simulation courses were to expose participants to the need for emergency training, to encourage use of checklists and cognitive aids, and to demonstrate the potential of simulation in training. The course was in no way a competency testing course, and lack of standardization in the course, lack of clear learning objectives, and lack of data collection were problematic. In addition, the operational model of the course in which a high facilitator-to-participant ratio was required and a knowledgeable simulator operator had to be available made the course expensive to run. The course was offered and operated at cost to the American Dental Society of Anesthesiology (cost neutral).

Parallel to this initial course was an ADA airway course, which was found to have similar problems. In 2007, the ADA Foundation put forth a request for proposals to medical and dental communities of interest, and in 2008 announced that Working Group of the Anesthesia Research Foundation of the American Dental Society of Anesthesiology, composed of Dr Daniel Becker, Dr Karen Crowley, Dr James Phero, and Dr Morton Rosenberg, was awarded a grant to develop an airway rescue course. Through pilot programs in Charleston, South Carolina, in 2008, and in Dayton, Ohio, in 2009, and proofs of concept in Las Vegas and Chicago in 2009, the project was completed and turned over to the ADA. The course consisted of a comprehensive monograph available in ADA CE online and a mandatory pretest. The hands-on portion included an orientation, standardized case scenarios, task training, multiple case scenarios, and a post-test. Formalized assessment was conducted for each participant, but the assessments lacked objective performance assessment criteria, and data collection was not possible. Besides the introduction of high-fidelity human simulation, other educational innovations included the use of the RespiTrainer (IngMar Medical) to quantitatively measure precourse and postcourse ventilatory parameters using a BMV and the Recording Resusci Anne simulator (Laerdal Medical) for basic CPR. The ADA course was presented at several locales over the years and the materials were available to appropriate

parties through the ADA. Unfortunately, despite a good basic effort, the course was not cost sustaining and had to be discontinued after several years.

DEVELOPMENT OF THE NEW SIMULATION PROGRAM

The AAOMS wanted to improve office-based anesthesia safety and develop a new simulation course that would complement the OAE process. The AAOMS sought to collaborate with a group with expertise in simulation training to create a simulation experience where participants could be trained to competency and tested on knowledge and hands-on skill and data collected and reported to prove the effectiveness of the training. The model needed to be cost sustaining and easily delivered across the country in a standardized manner (quality assurance and generalizability). Dr John Schaefer (Professor of Anesthesiology with an endowed chair) at the Medical University of South Carolina (MUSC) was consulted. Dr Schaefer's program, Health Care Simulation of South Carolina (HCSSC), and spin-off company, SimTunes, developed and deployed simulation educational and operational processes that included the simulation characteristics: (1) automated objective assessment, (2) high-volume, low-cost operational processes, (3) standardization of simulation delivery processes, and (4) multisite data recording and reporting. HCSSC had helped start or restart 30 health care simulation programs across the South Carolina tristate area. Its collaborative 14 sites were performing more than 100,000 simulations per year, including high-stakes courses tied to hospital physician procedural privileging process.

The CAN and MUSC developed 3 course modules: the basic emergency airway management course (BEAM), the office-based crisis management (OBCM) course, and the intravenous (IV) sedation course. The course was initially designed to be available to residency programs with an eventual expansion to simulation centers where an OMS could take staff to verify core competencies and correct deficiencies. It is also anticipated that if feasible, the course could be delivered from regional centers directly to practice locals. The AAOMS believed that the BEAM course was the highest patient safety priority and pursued that course as the initial program to be developed. As a result of the course, it is widely accepted and backed by closed claims data from the OMS National Insurance Company that airway urgencies and emergencies are the most common problem in high morbidity and mortality adverse events in OMS anesthesia and dental anesthesia. The BEAM course was designed to place emphasis on BMV rescue, because approximately 90% to 95% of airway urgencies can be initially managed with effective BMV.

The design of the program included self-paced, Internet-based, precourse didactic material and online video instruction; required a low facilitator-to-participant ratio (1 facilitator to 8 participants to 4 high-fidelity simulators; see **Fig. 1**) and software programming such that the participants could run the practice portion of the simulation program themselves with facilitator oversight; automatic objective testing for most elements; and a mastery-based cooperative learning model. The cooperative learning model is a model in which small groups work together in dyads to help each other learn material more efficiently than with other models. In the course, participants alternate roles to learn to perform skills, observe the primary learner, and operate the simulator. Each role allows for learning opportunities, and course learning criteria define success for skills.

Mastery-based learning involves practicing hands-on skills until objective performance criteria are met. In this approach, various methods are used:

- Mastery-based practice (MBP) is combined with progressive difficulty, which starts as easy for the novice and then becomes more difficult as learning progresses.
- Over-training, in which trainees practice beyond passing only once to enhance memory
- Adaptive learning that allows efficient progression of participants who meet training criteria early

Automatic performance data collection, feedback, and reporting are integrated into preprogrammed simulator scenarios (SimDesigner [Laerdal]) designed to be extremely easy to operate, such that participants can operate their own high-fidelity simulators (running these preprogrammed scenarios), requiring minimal training of less than 7 minutes to support cooperative learning and lower operational cost goals, given that fewer expert simulation support personnel are needed than for previous course approaches.

After a supervised MBP period, summative objective assessment is performed by the facilitator of each individual incorporating both technical and nontechnical performance metric criteria. If needed, remediation is achieved until all participants meet summative standards. The testing is high stakes and low risk in that although participants might not meet objective course standards, through MBP with remediation opportunities, all participants pass (to date within 2 post-test attempts). Once validated, the goal of the program is to create a data-driven and validated competency course similar to commercial aviation simulation. The course objectives for the BEAM course are listed in **Box 3** and the activities are shown in **Box 4**. The learning outcome measurements are shown in **Boxes 5–7**.

The principles for delivery of this program long term are to include a didactic online component and hands-on component and to standardize outcomes objectives. The programs must be validated over time through educational research and be regionally or locally available as well as cost sustainable and affordable. Value to participants lies in training for office-based emergencies and critical skill sets that are tightly coupled to

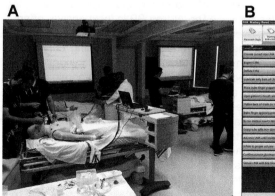
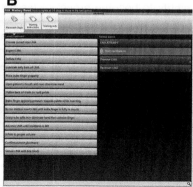

Fig. 1. (*A*) Training logistics of 1 facilitator to 4 high-fidelity simulators to 8 participants, with (*B*) participants operating simulators after 5 minutes of training using simple-to-operate preprogrammed scenarios.

Box 3
Basic emergency airway management course simulation training objectives: concepts and skills review

○ Sedation monitoring

○ Supplemental O_2 techniques

○ Techniques for opening the airway

○ BMV using 1-person and 2-person technique for normal and difficult mask airway[a]

○ Proper LMA insertion

○ Proper Airtraq technique

○ Appropriate treatment of mild, moderate, and severe laryngospasm in simulated adult and pediatric patients

[a] The difficult airway is mimicked by an airway restrictor device in the in the simulation mannequin, which has been tested and validated.[9]

Box 4
Basic emergency airway management course activities schedule

• Introduction—background, objective, overview, approach, and purpose.

• BEAM guidelines and card review

• Airway monitoring—key points and demonstration scenario

• Supplemental O_2 techniques

• Setting up O_2 tank, video demonstration, and exercise

• Nasal cannula review

• Face masks review

• Opening the airway techniques

• Triple airway maneuver—key points, demonstration, exercise

• Oral pharyngeal airway and nasal pharyngeal airway

• Bag-mask ventilation (BMV)

• One person, 2 persons, and video demonstration

• Simulation with mastery-based training (MBT) and assessment for 1 person, 2 persons, and difficult, with data collection

• LMA (LMA Unique, teleflex, US)

• Review, video demonstration, simulation, and MBT and assessment and data collection

• Airtraq video laryngoscope intubation

• Review, video demonstration, simulation MBT, and assessment and data collection

• Laryngospasm—review diagnosis, review treatment, group skills adult, and pediatric

---

historical closed claims–driven patient safety risks. The office team must take the course not only as individual practitioners but also as a team, because the course is designed to provide base critical individual and team-driven skills to manage office-based emergencies.

The BEAM course's content has been thoughtfully put together to best fill the needs of OMSs and OMS staff. First, it has been recognized that most of the adverse events in dental anesthesia are primarily respiratory in nature, resulting in the outline of the program. Second, although basic in some of its elements, it is designed for team training in which simple tasks, including assembling an O_2 tank, are included so all participants have a firm foundation of skills. During the pilot program, less than 25% of participants had ever assembled an O_2 tank during residency. De-emphasized is endotracheal intubation, a skill that requires a high number of practice attempts to become proficient (as high as 50) and one that deteriorates quickly over time without reinforcement. These facts, along with the knowledge that most airway emergencies can be managed with effective BMV, led the authors to emphasize this training with a supraglottic airway as the next step in management with a few exceptions. The laryngeal mask airway (LMA) was chosen as the supraglottic airway of choice because considerable literature was available demonstrating effectiveness, because of the low number of attempts to become proficient, and because of its easy teaching on simulators. Lastly, the Airtraq SP (Prodol Meditec, Getxo, Spain) was selected as

the video laryngoscope of choice for the course. Like supraglottic airways, there are many choices of video laryngoscope available for selection. The Airtraq SP is inexpensive, offers a variety of sizes, has a long shelf-life, and has support for its much shorter learning curve (3 to 5 intubations) than traditional laryngoscopy (30 to 50 intubations). The laryngospasm drills were performed as a small group exercise with 1 surgeon as team leader. Four different larygospasm scenarios were presented so each participant could train as team leader.

The pilots for the BEAM course were conducted at OMS residency programs at MUSC, University of Pittsburgh, University of Cincinnati, and University of Minnesota. For the pilot courses, residency training programs were used, and residents who had completed their training programs were

---

Box 5
Learning outcome measurements for normal and difficult bag-mask ventilation

- Overall BMV score (P/F)
- OPTIONAL placed an oral airway? (Y/N)
- OPTIONAL placed a nasal airway? (Y/N)
- Required a second person to assist? (Y/N)
- Oxygenation scores (time in range min:s):
  - Sao_2 above 98:
  - Sao_2 95 to 97:
  - Sao_2 92 to 94:
  - Sao_2 90 to 91:
  - Sao_2 89 or below:
- Ventilation scores (min:s):
  - Hyperventilation period: RR 16 or greater: RR 13 to 15:
  - Correct ventilation period: RR 9 to 12:
  - Hypoventilation period: RR 6 or less:
- TOTAL TRIALS COMPLETED to meet MBP criteria (min:s):

Abbreviations: BMV, bag-mask ventilation; P/F, pass/fail; RR, respiratory rate; Y/N, yes/no.

Box 6
Learning outcome measurements for laryngeal mask airway and Airtraq airway management skill

- Successful placement (Y/N):
- Number of steps correct:
- % Steps correct:
- Time to establish ventilations (min:s):
- Time to complete attempt (min:s):
- Steps missed or performed incorrectly (list of step[s]):
- Nontechnical score
  - Ready to perform on actual patient
  - Requires additional self-practice
  - Needs fundamental retraining of procedure by facilitator
- TOTAL TRIALS COMPLETED to meet MBP criteria:
- Total time to meet MBP criteria:

Box 7
Learning outcome measurements for adult and pediatric laryngospasm treatment drills

- OVERALL SCORE:
- GRADED STEPS COMPLETED:
- CRITICAL STEPS COMPLETED:
- Graded steps (correct or incorrect):
- TIME (MIN:S):
  - Available in drill:
  - Drill completed in:
  - Remaining in drill:
  - Removed stimulus:
  - Opened airway:
  - Administered succinylcholine (effective dose):
  - Administered propofol:

---

curves, training outcomes, and course quality assurance. A participant course survey was completed by each participant and logged into the software automatically.

The OBCM course, also known as CTT, is currently under development. A proof-of-concept pilot has been conducted, but the core material has not yet been completed at the time of this writing. One proof-of-concept pilot testing the methodology of the simulation has been conducted. The methodology and approach were new and had never been tested for feasibility. The design of the simulation was developed around 4-person teams, each with a specific role and specific goals to perform in a particular emergency. **Box 8** lists the roles for the oral and maxillofacial (OMF) office crisis team. As for the BEAM, the approach for emergency response for the OBCM was based on referenced best practices, and a set of support aids (cognitive aids) specific to each role was developed to facilitate overall team performance by predefining and organizing tasks related to the emergency.

Like the BEAM course, the OBCM will include an online course and a simulation workshop. The OBCM simulation training takes advantage of a new "multi-operator" feature of the simulator operating system software that supports the ability of having multiple operators adding input to the control of the software from networked PCs. As applied for OBCM training of a 4 person office team, it was used to both support "co-operative learning" as well as the quality benefits of team grading with four observers rather than one

selected. Examples of sample data are shown in **Figs. 2–5**. A table of data collected is shown in **Box 7**. Each pilot generated approximately 8000 data points, which can be used to analyze learning

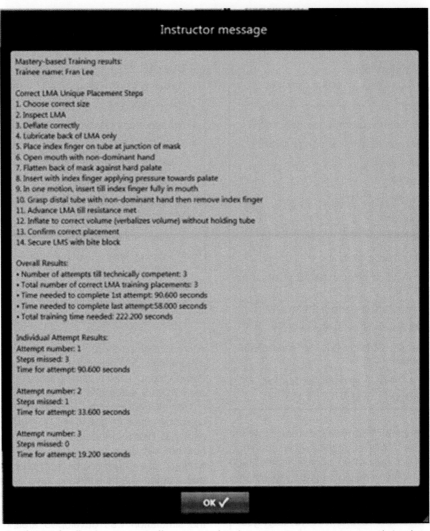

Fig. 2. Sample of MBP feedback automatically presented to learner using preprogrammed simulator scenario.

observer. Each training session involves two teams with one team (of 4 office healthcare givers) performing the training exercise and the second team has each team member observing their equivalent role on the first team using one of the networked PCs to record observed actions. At the end of the simulation exercise, the software automatically compiled grades & notes (scored against best practice protocols for a given emergency) reflecting both "overall" Team performance in context of patient care and outcome as well as individual breakdown of team members roles and tasks with how this impacted outcome (**Fig. 6**). Anaphylaxis was used as the emergency for the proof-of-concept pilot. Data were collected and aggregated, and through software development by SimTunes, the aggregate data can be collected

simultaneously. Criteria were developed that included high pass, marginal pass, good (pass), fail, and dangerous fail. In the scenario, the team had 8 minutes to complete all tasks before paramedics arrived. **Box 9** shows scoring criteria for the pilot program.

Based on the success of the proof-of-concept pilot for anaphylaxis, the AAOMS has contracted with SimTunes to design a simulation program that will include Internet-based modules and 4 team training exercises to hands-on practice with teams performing simulations. **Box 10** lists the components of the OBCM/CTT training. The IV sedation course is not yet developed and will be the third tier of the AAOMS simulation program. Likely an online training program rather than hands-on, the program will review concepts of IV

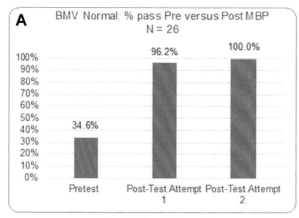
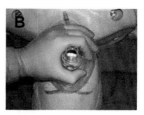
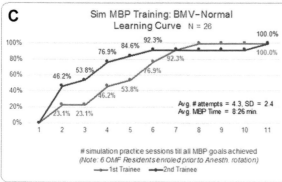
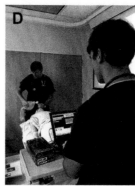

Fig. 3. Sample training outcomes for bag-mask ventilation training across 4 pilot sites (N = 26) using cooperative learning and MBP. (*A*) Delta of learning from beginning to end of MBT (% of all trainees who passed). (*B*) Picture of technique learned. (*C*) Learning curve data. (*D*) Trainee "co-operative learning" example with technique.

sedation for the office setting. It is envisioned that the program will allow for review of pharmacology, titration, and monitoring by using scenario-based learning with case presentations and case management online, with a vital signs monitor screen that would respond predictably with the inputs of the practitioner. Review of patients' medical history, selection for depth of sedation, selection of drugs, and drug dose responses can be programmed into the software. In this way, practitioners can become familiar with drugs and techniques not familiar to them in a realistic way and can gain experience without risk of patient harm.

SUMMARY

The AAOMS simulation program has been a multi-year effort to improve on patient safety in the office environment. The first part of this program, the BEAM course, is available for national distribution and as of this writing is scheduled for a train-the-trainer program to allow for development of

facilitators for distribution of the course. The OBCM/CTT program is currently under development with a tentative pilot date in early 2018.

The components of the simulation program will need to collect data, and the courses will need to be validated. Validation can be rated easily through several criteria, including

- Differentiation, meaning the course differentiates experienced practitioners from a novice group
- Educational goals, measured in the pretest and post-test phases of the course
- Inter-rater reliability, judging whether the course tests what it is supposed to test
- Translation, which asks if training in the course provides predictive validity and competency for trainees, that is, comparing a novice group with and without the course and their use of the LMA or Airtraq SP

There are obstacles ahead for the AAOMS simulation program: politics and proof of critical value exceeding training costs. Should the planned

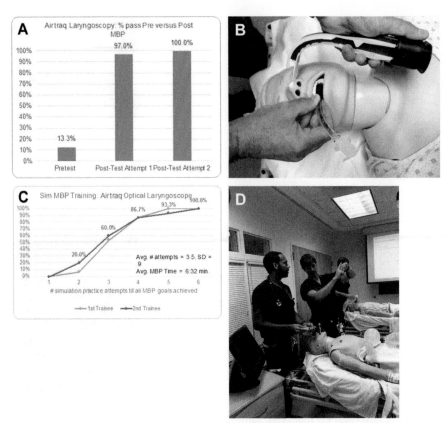

Fig. 4. Sample training outcomes for Airtraq intubation training across 4 pilot sites (N = 26) using cooperative learning and MBP. (*A*) Delta of learning from beginning to end of MBT (% of all trainees who passed). (*B*) Picture of technique learned. (*C*) Learning curve data. (*D*) Trainee "co-operative learning" example with technique.

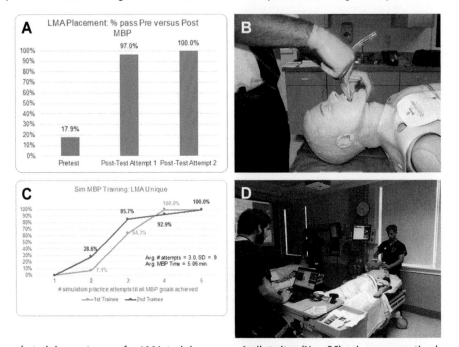

Fig. 5. Sample training outcomes for LMA training across 4 pilot sites (N = 26) using cooperative learning and MBP. (*A*) Delta of learning from beginning to end of MBT (% of all trainees who passed). (*B*) Picture of technique learned. (*C*) Learning curve data. (*D*) Trainee "co-operative learning" example with technique.

<table>
<tr><td>

Box 8
Base roles for oral and maxillofacial office–based crisis team

- OMF surgeon, team leader
- Assistant 1
- Assistant 2
- Team coordinator (circulator)

</td><td>

Box 9
Grading criteria for office-based crisis management team

- Perfect (high pass)
  - Time to ventilation <2 min; time to 911 call <2 min; time to Dx <2 min; administer Epi × 2, albuterol, fluids, diphenhydramine, methylprednisolone, and ranitidine
- Okay (marginal pass)
  - Time to ventilation <4 min; time to 911 call <4 min; time to diagnosis <4 min; administer epinephrine × 2, albuterol, and fluids
- Good (pass)
  - Any score between perfect and marginal pass
- Fail
  - Any score less than marginal pass
- Dangerous fail
  - Placed LMA, intubated, administered dangerous drug or did not administer drugs as ordered

</td></tr>
</table>

validation and predictive validity research prove true, the authors believe that the course should be mandated, and a time-limited certificate should be issued. Furthermore, state laws must change to include and require simulation training. The authors believe the program will be opposed by a vocal minority who will not want to have another mandate imposed on them. This is understandable, and concerns must be addressed through demonstration of valid, meaningful value to practices at the lowest costs practical. Cost is a significant concern, because simulation center costs generally are high with today's operational methods, and the program and equipment costs must be met. The current AAOMS course carries one-fourth the operational costs at 4 times the throughput of previous offerings, which promises a more practical per medical CE hour. Healthcare practitioners must do all they can improve patient safety—the public is becoming increasingly aware and sensitive to highly publicized adverse events, rare or not. The BEAM course and OBCM/CTT will offer objective assessment of practitioner and team competency and is an important step

assuring our patients, the public, and regulators that we can competently and safely perform office-based anesthesia and avoid or proficiently mitigate the potentially injurious events to our patients. That is the critical value that will outweigh the costs of training as it has in commercial aviation. Data-driven standardized simulation training

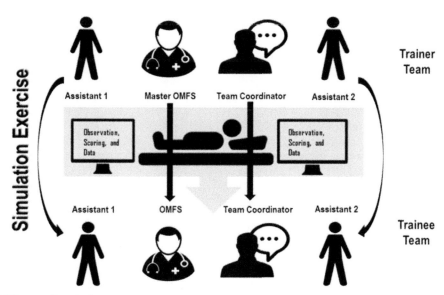

Fig. 6. OBCM operational schema.

> **Box 10**
> **Office-based crisis management/crisis team training course outline**
>
> - Internet-based curricula modules
>   - Anaphylaxis
>   - Respiratory arrest secondary to sedation
>   - Laryngospasm
>   - Negative pressure pulmonary edema
>   - Bronchospasm airway emergency
>   - Malignant hyperthermia
>   - Aspiration
>   - Cardiac chest pain
>   - Cardiac arrhythmia
>   - Local anesthetic systemic toxicity
> - Scenarios for applying the protocols, roles, goals, and processes
>   - Anaphylaxis (adult, severe)
>   - Laryngospasm (adult & pediatric, complete)
>   - Respiratory arrest secondary to sedation (adult, difficult BMV)
>   - Chest pain proceeding to arrhythmia (adult, hypertension, chest pain progresses to ventricular tachycardia)

is one of the pillars that forms the current public trust in commercial aviation safety. Similarly, the current AAOMS simulation training-based patient safety course project is a promising step down this path with the aim of seringe both patients and colleagues.

REFERENCES

1. Ritt RM, Bennett JD, Todd DW. Simulation training for the office-based anesthesia team. Oral Maxillofacial Surg Clin N Am 2017;29:169–78.
2. Park CS. Simulation and quality improvement in anesthesiology. Anesthesiol Clin 2011;29:13–28.
3. Cant RP, Cooper SJ. Simulation -based learning in nurse education: systematic review. J Adv Nurs 2010;66(1):3–15.
4. Schaefer JJ, Vanderbilt AA, Casan CL, et al. Literature review: instructional design and pedagogy science in healthcare simulation. Simul Healthc 2011;6:S30–41.
5. Issenberg SB, McGaghie WC, Petrusa ER, et al. Features and uses of high-fidelity medical simulations that lead to effective learning: a BEME systematic review. Med Teach 2005;27(1):10–28.
6. Maran NJ, Glavin RJ. Low to high-fidelity simulation – a continuum of medical education? Med Education 2003;37:22–8.
7. Draycott T, Sibanda T, Owen L, et al. Does training in obstetric emergencies improve neonatal outcome? BJOG 2006;113:177–82.
8. Draycott TJ, Crofts JF, Ash JP, et al. Improved outcomes after shoulder dystocia training. Obstet Gynecol 2008;112:14–20.
9. Pastis NJ, Doelken P, Vanderbilt AA, et al. Validation of Simulated Difficult Bag-Mask Ventilation as a Training and Evaluation Method for First-Year Internal Medicine House Staff. Journal of the Society for Simulation in Healthcare 2013;8(1).

Airway Management for the Oral Surgery Patient

Allan Schwartz, DDS, CRNA

KEYWORDS

- Airway • Airway assessment • Open airway oral surgery • Open system airway devices
- Closed airway oral surgery • Closed system airway devices • Airway emergencies • Aspiration

KEY POINTS

- Office-based oral surgery occurs in the head and the neck area and can occur in close proximity to the glottis. Both the establishment and maintenance of the airway during oral surgery are paramount and foremost to the success of the surgery.
- Preoperative airway assessment is key to a thorough history and physical examination. Dental facial profiles and certain oral characteristics and presentations are essential parts of tested anesthetic airway evaluation and valuable predictors of continuous airway patency throughout the oral surgical procedure.
- Extreme caution while performing oral, head, and neck procedures along with knowledge of currently available airway protection and maintenance devices are critical for oral surgical practice and should be available as part of an oral surgeon's airway arsenal.
- Open system and closed system airway devices are discussed. Devices are presented according to their level of invasiveness and discomfort to patients as well as the level of skill required of oral surgeons in their placement.
- Airway emergency intervention protocols are essential to patient care. The oral and maxillofacial surgery difficult airway algorithm is reviewed.

INTRODUCTION

The human airway is a complex of anatomic structures, acute angles, secretions, and powerful musculature. Human reflexes exquisitely and strongly guard and maintain the patency of the airway to prevent intrusion from foreign matter. Management of this small area is paramount and foremost to all successful office anesthesia outcomes. Safe anesthetic delivery is dependent on careful patient selection and airway management. This article serves as a guide and reference for oral surgeons in completing a preoperative airway history and airway physical examination using tested airway evaluation tools to screen for patients who likely are at risk for a difficult airway. This article also reviews the selection of the proper airway device to help in patient management. Lastly, an oral surgical airway emergency intervention algorithm is discussed.

MEDICAL HISTORY AND PHYSICAL EXAMINATION

An example of a thorough preoperative medical history is shown in Appendix 1.

After a thorough review of systems, exploration of airway-related questions is a necessity. Questions should pertain to history of difficulty with previous anesthetics, recent upper respiratory infections, asthma, shortness of breath, bronchitis, pneumonia, and chronic obstructive pulmonary

Dedication: This article could not have been accomplished without the help of Anita Schwartz; Leonard & Lita Schwartz; Carol Hoepner; Gary Clark, EdD, CRNA and the late Harvey Bloom, DDS.
Department of Periodontics, The Center for Advanced Dental Education, Saint Louis University, 3320 Rutger Street, St Louis, MO 63104, USA
E-mail address: sedationconsult@outlook.com

disease. Any history of snoring or obstructive sleep apnea and the use of continuous positive airway pressure are signs of probable difficult airway management as the level of sedation deepens. A STOP-Bang questionnaire can be useful for confirming likelihood of obstructive sleep apnea.

BASIC CLINICAL AIRWAY ANATOMY AND ASSESSMENT

Anesthesia providers routinely use several focused airway assessment tools and patient observations in combination when assessing a patient prior to anesthesia treatment.[1–9] All these airway assessment tools are based on dental oral and facial anatomic features. It is important to recognize that there are factors that predict difficulty of bag-valve-mask (BVM) ventilation and those that predict difficulty for intubation, and they are not the same lists (**Box 1**). When performing patient selection for office-based anesthesia, choosing patients who can be successfully ventilated with a BVM is desired because this airway management procedure resolves the vast majority of airway urgencies. It is also important that use of an airway when performing BVM increases the chance of success greatly. Choosing patients who can be predictably intubated if that need arises in an emergency is also desired.

Box 1
Factors predicting difficulty with bag-valve-mask

Age greater than 55

Body mass index greater than 26

Edentulism

Presence of a beard

History of snoring

Active airway obstruction (abscess, tumor, edema)

   Factors predicting difficulty with intubation

High Mallampati class

Retrognathia

Short thyromental distance

Limited interincisal distance

Restricted range of motion of the neck

Severe obesity

Upper lip bite test class II or class II

The tucking of the tongue into a space down and away from the isthmus of the fauces into the floor of the mouth is essential during intubation. The depth and width of the throat and pharynx necessitate observing the uvula, the soft palate, and the extension of the tongue.

The following is a list of some commonly used chairside noninvasive patient airway assessment tools. Preoperative airway assessment should be documented in the patient record.

Mallampati Classification

First proposed in 1983,[10] Seshagiri Mallampati, MD, and colleagues published an article in 1985, entitled, "A Clinical Sign To Predict Difficult Tracheal Intubation; A Prospective Study" in the *Journal of the Canadian Anaesthesia Society* (**Fig. 1**).[11] His name is synonymous with a quick preoperative study of the possibility for airway difficulty and maintenance for anesthetic patients.[1,4–7,10–15]

Mallampati examination is performed by laying a patient nearly supine, with the head placed on a pillow and the neck extended into the sniffing position. The patient is then asked to open the mouth as wide as possible and protrude the tongue. The procedure should be performed without vocalization.[5,16] A wide intermaxillary distance is a key necessity for performing any intraoral assessments and is especially important for visualization and purchase of the airway during anesthesia.[17] Temporomandibular joint range of motion is related to this assessment.

Mallampati initially proposed 3 airway assessment classifications. The fourth classification was included for patients who showed no view of the base of the uvula with only the view soft palate on maximum mouth opening with tongue protrusion. Also, a Mallampati class 0 airway was proposed by Ezri and colleagues[18] in 2001. With a Mallampati class 0 airway, the tip of the epiglottis is viewed while performing the assessment.[18,19]

Angle External Facial Profile Classifications

Edward Angle, DDS, known as the "Father of Modern Orthodontics," proposed a classification of external facial profiles. His research and teaching described 3 facial profiles that patients could exhibit when viewing the face from a lateral position. Each of these profiles can reflect an undersized or oversized mandible for placement of the tongue as well as position of the teeth and other facial bony structures.

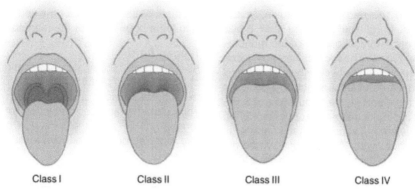

Fig. 1. Samsoon classification system. The oropharynx is divided into 4 classes on the basis of the structures visualized: class I—soft palate, fauces, uvula, pillars; class II—soft palate, fauces, uvula; class III—soft palate, base of uvula; and class IV—soft palate not visible. (*From* Mallampati SR. Recognition of the difficult airway. In: Benumof JL, editor. Airway management: principles and practice. St Louis (MO): Mosby; 1996. p. 132; with permission.)

Angle class I—orthognathic profile

Angle described the orthognathic profile as the mesiobuccal cusp of the maxillary first molar aligned with the mesiobuccal groove of the mandibular first molar (**Fig. 2**). When viewing the patient profile laterally, the cephalometric points of the glabella, nasion, and menton form a relatively straight line. This can indicate probable ease of both tucking the tongue and visualizing the laryngeal inlet.

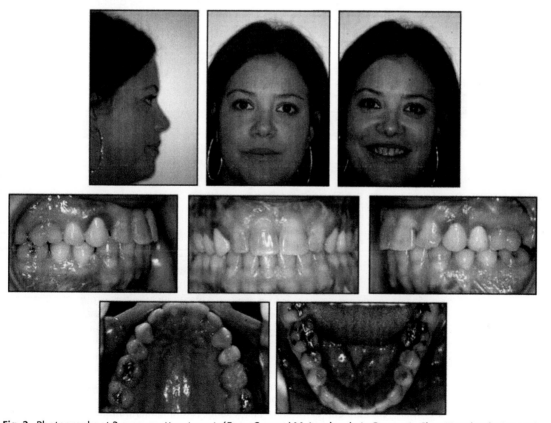

Fig. 2. Photographs at 2 years posttreatment. (*From* Cozzani M, Lombardo L, Gracco A. Class III malocclusion with missing maxillary lateral incisors. Am J Orthod Dentofacial Orthop 2011;139:395; with permission.)

Angle class II—retrognathic profile

Angle described the retrognathic profile as the mesiobuccal cusp of the maxillary first molar mesial to the mesiobuccal groove of the mandibular first molar (**Fig. 3**). The menton is a point posterior to the line formed between the glabella and nasion. The result is usually a lack of space for tucking into the floor of the mouth due to the relaxed tongue musculature produced during sedation. An extreme version of this profile is seen in the patient with Pierre-Robin syndrome, Treacher-Collins syndrome, or Nager syndrome.[14]

Angle class III—prognathic profile

Angle described the prognathic profile as the mesiobuccal cusp of the maxillary first molar distal to the mesiobuccal groove of the mandibular first molar (**Fig. 4**). The menton is anterior to the line formed by the glabella and the nasion. This is a favorable profile for airway control prediction because of the large area provided for the tongue within the boundaries of the mandible.

Tongue tuck

As described in the Angle classifications, a patient can be taught to perform a tongue tuck, by pulling the tongue inferiorly and posteriorly[20,21] (**Fig. 5**). This demonstrates a prediction of where the tongue will lie after the induction of anesthesia and muscle paralysis for laryngoscopy.

Thyromental Distance

Thyromental distance is an important airway assessment tool that is mentioned as an important adjunct in conjunction with several other airway assessment tools in the literature (**Fig. 6**).[3,4,6,12,14,15,22] Thyromental distance is

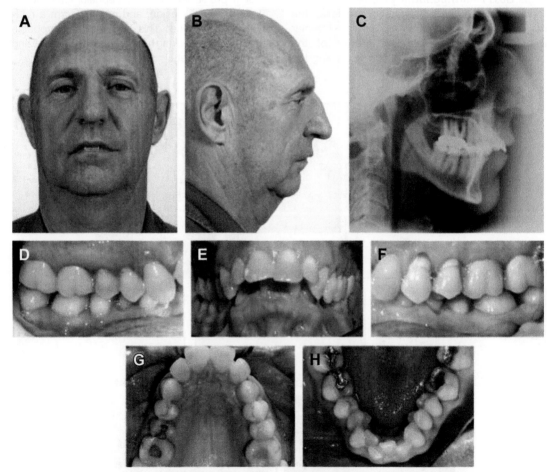

Fig. 3. Frontal facial (*A*), lateral facial (*B*), lateral cephalometric (*C*), and intraoral (*D–H*) pretreatment images of 59-year-old man with severe obstructive sleep apnea (apnea-hypopnea index = 45), decreased posterior airway space, and concomitant maxillofacial skeletal deformities (mandibular retrognathia, transverse maxillary hypoplasia, and transverse mandibular hypoplasia). (*From* Boyd SB. Management of obstructive sleep apnea by maxillomandibular advancement. Oral Maxillofac Surg Clin North Am 2009;21:450; with permission.)

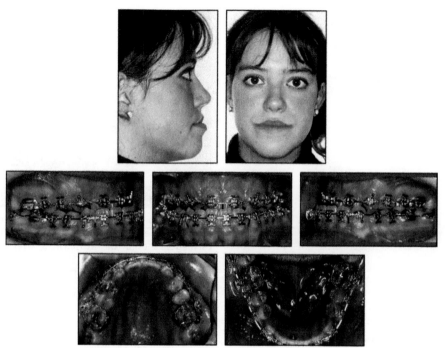

Fig. 4. Leveling and alignment. (*From* Cozzani M, Lombardo L, Gracco A. Class III malocclusion with missing maxillary lateral incisors. Am J Orthod Dentofacial Orthop 2011;139:395; with permission.)

the distance, measured in fingerbreadths, from the orthognathic menton point or the protuberance of the mentum to the superior portion of the thyroid cartilage when viewed laterally. This assessment tool is related to the Angle assessment, described previously. Thyromental distance is an easily performed assessment and provides yet another means of documenting the length of the mandible.

Dental Protrusion or Flare

The natural or exaggerated outward angle of the maxillary and/or the mandibular anterior teeth can potentially interfere with intubation due to the fixed length of laryngoscope blades (**Fig. 7**). Flare can also be caused by advanced periodontal disease. Mobility of periodontally involved anterior teeth can lead to potential dental damage and/or dislodgment of teeth with the potential for dental damage, tooth swallowing, or tooth aspiration.

Diastema

A wide maxillary anterior midline diastema can interfere with the placement of a MacIntosh laryngoscope blade whose vertical portion could catch or fall in between the diastema[23] (**Fig. 8**). Lip trauma can also occur due to the lifting forces applied during laryngoscopy causing the maxillary lip to fall traumatically into the diastema.

Total Edentulism

The absence of teeth in the maxillary and mandibular arches can provide relative ease for visualizing airway structures and thus enable easier placement of an endotracheal tube (ETT) or supraglottic airway, such as the laryngeal mask airway (LMA) or King Airway (KA [King Systems Corporation, Ballerup, Denmark]) (**Fig. 9**). Patients who are totally edentulous, however, are more difficult to mask ventilate.

Full-Arch Fixed-Dental Prostheses

The fragility of all ceramic tooth prostheses and porcelain fused to metal prostheses necessitates the slow and careful navigation of airway devices and laryngoscope blades into proper position for direct laryngoscopy (**Fig. 10**A). Dental damage is a minor but costly cause of lawsuits by patients during airway manipulation according to closed claim data from the American Society of Anesthesiologists.[24–27]

Dental Arch Tooth Protector

A disposable rubberized plastic tooth protector is available to cover fixed-dental prostheses and natural teeth during laryngoscopy (**Fig. 10**B). Use of a video laryngoscope, such as an Airtraq (Airtraq Corporation, Miami, FL), inserted intraorally along the midline, allows lesser manipulation of dental

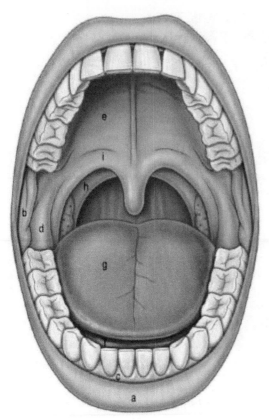

Fig. 5. The oral cavity consists of the lips (a), buccal mucosa (b), mandibular and maxillary alveolar ridge (c), retromolar trigone (d), hard palate (e), floor of the mouth (f), and oral tongue (g). The main structures in the oral pharynx are the base of the tongue, tonsillar pillars (h), lateral and posterior pharyngeal walls, and soft palate (i). (*From* Yu P. Intraoral, pharynx, and cervical esophagus. In: Butler CE, editor. Head and neck reconstruction. Philadelphia: Saunders; 2009. p. 167–96; with permission.)

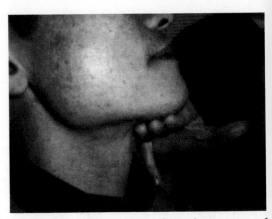

Fig. 6. Thyromental distance (from the mentum of the mandible to the upper margin of the thyroid cartilage) should be at least 3 average fingerbreadths. (*From* Orebaugh SL. Definition, incidence, and predictors of the difficult airway. In: Atlas of airway management: techniques and tools. Philadelphia: Lippincott Williams & Wilkins; 2007. p. 45; with permission.)

tissues compared with traditional metal laryngoscopes along with a reduced amount of force necessary to uncover and view the glottis. Careful manipulation of airway devices and equipment in this potentially fragile dental restorative environment requires additional time compared with natural and unrestored dental tissues. This increased time requirement can be costly when confronted with a difficult airway. Obese patients can especially quickly deoxygenate with a profound rapid drop in oxygen saturation due to their decreased functional residual capacity.

Narrow Palatal Arch Width

Placement of supraglottic airway devices and laryngoscopy equipment can be impaired when there is reduced space for manipulation of the device (**Fig. 11**). Visualization can also be impaired due to this narrowing of space.

Bony and Soft Tissue Obstructions (Palatal and Mandibular Tori; Oral Masses)

Bony obstructions of the mandible can impede the space needed for the tucking of the tongue for placement of airway devices and equipment (**Fig. 12**). Oral masses can interfere with visualizations of the airway as well as be a friable source of bleeding.

Head and Neck Range of Motion

Voluntary movement of the head and neck should always be a part of a thorough airway examination[6,17] (**Fig. 13**). The patient is asked to carefully rotate the head to its full comfortable extent in an extended position, flexed position, a right lateral turn, and then a left lateral turn. Then, have the patient extend the head and neck into the sniffing position while keeping the shoulders rested against the dental chair. This is especially important for elderly patients who may have arthritis of their cervical vertebrae or patients who have had cervical spine surgery.

Previous Tracheostomy

Surgical intervention for a tracheostomy can leave a scarred and stenotic glottis that can interfere with the passage of an ETT past the glottic inlet (**Figs. 14** and **15**). Have a variety of smaller-diameter cuffed ETTs available.

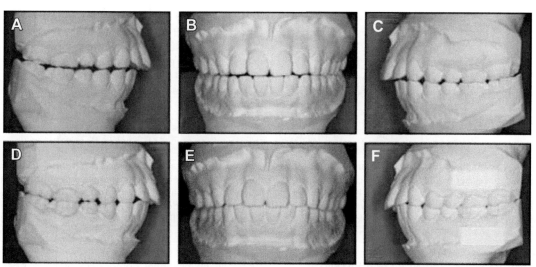

Fig. 7. Dental casts mounted in centric relation: (*A–C*) class II molar and canine relationships and large overjet and open bite were observed; (*D–F*) occlusal adjustment of the casts to close the bite confirms the extent of the class II occlusion and excess overjet. (*From* Nelson G, Ahn HW, Jeong SH, et al. Three-dimensional retraction of anterior teeth with orthodontic miniplates in patients with temporomandibular disorder. Am J Orthod Dentofacial Orthop 2012;142:720; with permission.)

Periodontal Disease and Dental Caries Status

Carious and periodontally involved teeth can provide a multitude of potential serious airway difficulties due to tooth and calculus fragments, tooth fractures, tooth luxation, mobility, and hemorrhage (**Fig. 16**).

Upper Lip Bite Test

The upper lip bite test demonstrates the range of motion of the mandible in both rotational and translational movements[2,4,14,28,29] (**Fig. 17**). These same movements are performed during laryngoscopy.

Reduced Muscle Strength or Weakness

Reduced muscle strength or weakness can lead to dislocation of the mandible during laryngoscopy.[30]

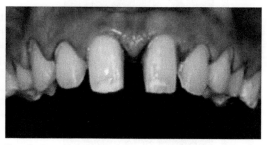

Fig. 8. Preparations to try to mesialize teeth and move dental midline to the patient's left. (*From* Calamia V. Simple case treatment planning. Dent Clin North Am 2015;59:660; with permission.)

Quick recognition of the dislocation followed by relocation of the mandible while the patient is deeply anesthetized or pharmacologically paralyzed is necessary.

Airway Assessment Guide

The airway assessment guide visually summarizes the airway assessment tools, described previously. It may be downloaded from this Web address: https://www.sedationconsult.com/store/p112/Clinical_Airway_Assessment_Guide.html.

PATIENT POSITIONING

Position the patient preoperatively using feedback regarding comfort to prevent skin breakdown from contact pressures caused by equipment. Be cognizant of proper patient positioning for adequate circulation, padding of bony prominences, patient warmth, head and neck position, and the use of clear lens protective goggles or eye tape for prevention of corneal abrasion. For prolonged oral surgical procedures, consider the possibility of venous thromboembolism developing in a sedentary patient. The oral surgeon or assistant can manipulate the legs by lifting them individually above the level of the heart and gently massaging the tissues, moving venous blood back toward the central circulation. Sequential compression devices are available and inexpensive and can be used for patients at high risk for venous thromboembolism.

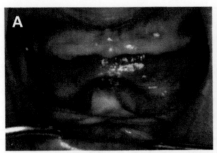
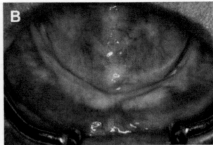

Fig. 9. Loss of the alveolar ridge in an edentulous patient brings the mental foramen and the inferior alveolar nerve canal closer to the surface, which may lead to discomfort for the patient. (*A*) Anterior view demonstrating a severe loss of vertical alveolar ridge height. (*B*) Occlusal view of the same patient demonstrating a loss of vestibular depth with alveolar bone loss. (*From* Carranza FA, Klokkevold PR. Periodontal and periimplant surgical anatomy. In: Newman MG, Takei HH, Klokkevold PR, et al, editors. Carranza's clinical periodontolgy. St Louis (MO): Saunders; 2015. p. 557–65; with permission.)

CLINICAL MAINTENANCE OF A PATENT AIRWAY

Sniffing Position

The sniffing position is the ideal position for the maintenance of the airway during sedation (**Fig. 18**).

Ramping

Ramping is the judicious use of blankets, towels, cervical pillows, and foam supports, which physically positions the obese and morbidly obese patient for bag-mask ventilation and laryngoscopy (**Figs. 19–21**). It is performed by placing supports so that the mastoid process and the sternum are at the same level. It is not an ideal working position, however, except for access to the maxillary arch.

Triple Airway Maneuver

The triple airway maneuver consists of heat tilt/chin lift, jaw thrust, and opening the mouth and is used as an essential component of head positioning to open the airway (**Fig. 22**).

Jaw Thrust

Forceful anterior translation of the mandible is an extremely stimulating maneuver and can counteract the level of sedation required for the surgical procedure (**Fig. 23**).

Throat Pack

Because oral surgical procedures involve an open (entrainment of some amount of room air) airway with unsecured access to the glottis and the trachea, the throat pack acts as a physical barrier and protection against the entry of foreign substances toward the laryngeal inlet. The closed system surgical throat pack is shown in **Fig. 24**A, B, whereas the open system surgical throat pack is shown in **Fig. 24**C.

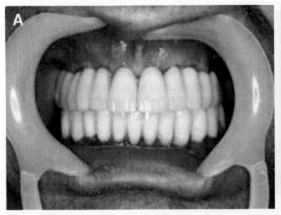
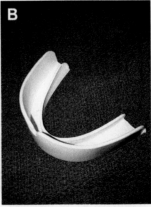

Fig. 10. (*A*) Final full-arch fixed-dental prostheses. (*B*) Dental arch tooth protector. (*From* Altintas NY, Taskesen F, Bagis B, et al. Immediate implant placement in fresh sockets versus implant placement in healed bone for full-arch fixed prostheses with conventional loading. Int J Oral Maxillofac Surg 2016;45:227; with permission.)

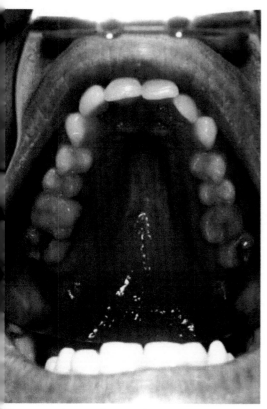

Fig. 11. An intraoral view of a patient with a high, narrow palate. (*From* Guyuron B. Correcting deviated noses, septoplasty and turbinectomy. In: Rhinoplasty. Philadelphia: Saunders; 2012. p. 311; with permission.)

AIRWAY MANAGEMENT DEVICES FOR ORAL SURGERY

Airway management consists of a continuum of 3 possible interventions in the perioperative period. If a patient is sedated and has an open airway and is hypoventilating, oxygen may simply have to be supplemented with a nasal cannula or face mask. If a patient's own ventilatory effort is not sufficient, ventilations may have to be assisted with Bag mask ventilation. If a patient is deeply sedated or is undergoing a general anesthetic, ventilations may have to be controlled with BVM, supraglottic airway, or ETT.

Oral Pharyngeal Airway (Berman Airway or Guedel Airway)

The oral pharyngeal airway (OPA) can only be placed once gag reflexes are lost but can be a quickly inserted and efficient device for the establishment and maintenance of the airway in an obtunded patient. The contour of the OPA approximates the shape of the human airway and can have either a hollow central portion or lateral tracks to allow the flow of fresh gas. An OPA is sized by siting the distance between the angle of the mandible and the commissure of the mouth.

Nasal Pharyngeal Airway or Nasal Trumpet

The nasal pharyngeal airway (NPA) or Nasal Trumpet is sized by siting the distance between the ala of the nose and the tragus of the ear. The NPA is lubricated with a water-soluble lubricant and inserted into the narae with gentle pressure parallel to the plane of the hard palate and a right/left twisting motion. The curvature of the NPA guides itself posteriorly toward the superior area of the nasopharynx. Copious nose bleeding can occur with the NPA despite gentle insertion technique. Consider spraying the nare generously with an oxymetazoline-containing nasal spray (Afrin) prior to insertion.

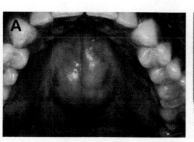
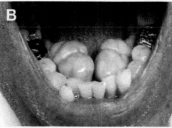
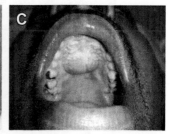

Fig. 12. (*A*) Torus palatinus. Midline bony nodule of the palatal vault. (*B*) Mandibular tori. (*C*) Midline palatal swelling. The symmetry and anatomic location of the mass should be noted. (*From* [A] Neville B, Damm DD, Allen CM, et al. Developmental defects of the oral and maxillofacial region. In: Oral and maxillofacial pathology. St Louis (MO): Elsevier; 2016. p. 1–48, with permission; and [B] Swartz MH. The oral cavity and pharynx. In: Textbook of physical diagnosis: history and examination. 7th ed. Philadelphia, PA: Elsevier; 2014. p. 278-314; with permission; and [C] Manzon S, Graffeo M, Philbert R. Median palatal cyst: case report and review of literature. J Oral Maxillofac Surg 2009;67:927, with permission.)

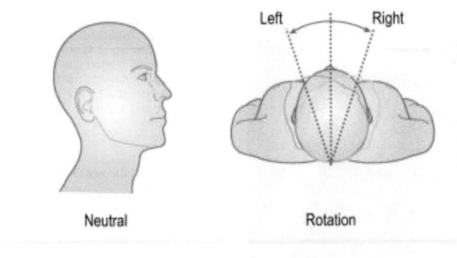

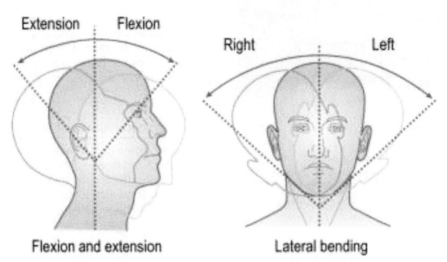

Fig. 13. Movements of the neck. (*From* D'Cruz DP. Locomotor system. In: Glynn M, Drake WM, editors. Hutchison's clinical methods: an integrated approach to clinical practice. Philadelphia: Saunders; 2012. p. 249–82; with permission.)

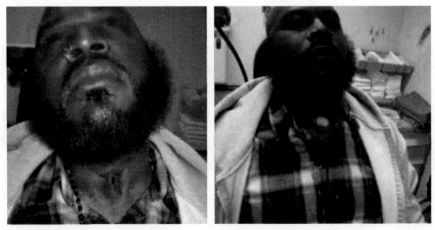

Fig. 14. Permanent tracheostomy. (*From* Maisel RH, Yang RZ. Permanent but reversible tracheostomy for severe symptomatic obstructive sleep apnea. Operative Techniques in Otolaryngology: Head and Neck Surgery 2015;26:204; with permission.)

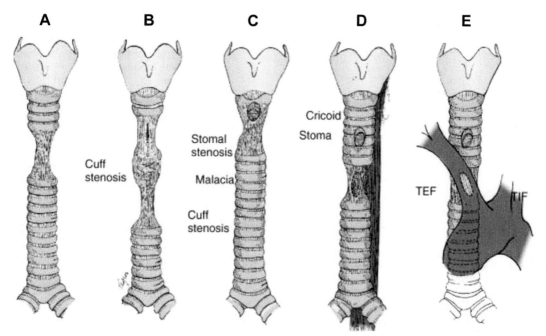

A   **B**   **C**   **D**   **E**

Cuff
stenosis

Stomal
stenosis

Malacia

Cuff
stenosis

Cricoid

Stoma

TEF

TIF

Fig. 15. Diagrams of principal postintubation tracheal lesions. (*A*) Cuff stenosis from the cuff of an ETT. (*B*) Cuff stenosis from the cuff of a tracheostomy tube, usually lower in the trachea than that from an ETT. Stoma stenosis also occurs at the site of the tracheostomy itself. Malacia can occur either at the level of the cuff or in the segment between the stoma and the cuff stenosis. (*C*) Cuff stenosis at the site of a high tracheostomy stoma, which has eroded into the lower margin of the cricoid cartilage. In older patients, this can erode back further into the sub-glottic larynx, producing a laryngotracheal stenosis. (*D*) Tracheoesophageal fistula (TEF) produced by pressure of the cuff against the membranous wall, often abetted by an indwelling, firm, nasogastric tube. (*E*) One type of tracheoinnominate fistula (TIF) is the result of a high-pressure cuff erosion. The more common type, but also rare, is that seen with a low-placed tracheostomy stoma, which rests against the innominate artery itself. Not shown here are the lesions that occur in the larynx as the result of ETTs. (*From* Grillo HC. Surgical management of postintubation tracheal injuries. J Thorac Cardiovasc Surg 1979;78:860; with permission.)

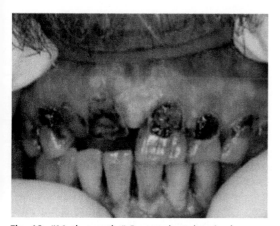

Fig. 16. "Meth mouth." Severe dental caries because of methamphetamine abuse. (*From* Hamamoto DT, Rhodus NL. Methamphetamine abuse and dentistry. Oral Dis 2009;15:27–37; with permission.)

Laryngeal Mask Airway

The supraglottic device, LMA, forms a seal above the laryngeal inlet. Once the LMA is deeply inserted into the posterior pharynx, it is inflated with air to help seal the mask portion within the supraglottic portion of the airway. The LMA is available in a full range of sizes. The LMA Supreme (LMA North America, San Diego, CA) contains a curve to ease insertion of the device and also contains a bite block to prevent collapse of the gas delivery tube from clenching during emergence. The LMA Supreme also contains a lumen through its center to allow the passage of a 26-French orogastric tube to facilitate the evacuation of liquid gastric contents. The LMA Flexible is an LMA with a wire reinforced flexible airway tube allowing it to be retracted without dislodging the seal of the LMA in the oral pharynx.

LMA Fastrach

The LMA Fastrach (LMAF, Fatraq Corporation, Eagan, MN) is a specialized reusable LMA

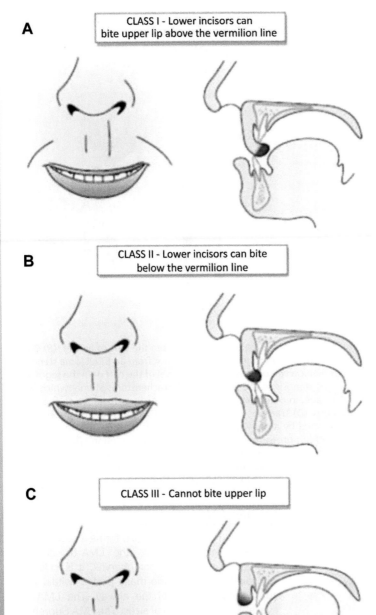

A CLASS I - Lower incisors can bite upper lip above the vermilion line

B CLASS II - Lower incisors can bite below the vermilion line

C CLASS III - Cannot bite upper lip

Fig. 17. The upper lip bite test. (*From* Khan Z, Kashif A, Ebrahimkhani E. A comparison of the upper lip bite test (a simple new technique with modified Mallampati classification in predicting difficulty in endotracheal intubation: a prospective blinded study. Anesth Analg 2003:96:596–7; with permission.)

consisting of 4 components: a curved LMAF mask portion with a metal handle to help firmly grasp the LMA for insertion, a special LMAF wire-reinforced 6.0-mm inner-diameter ETT (LMAF ETT), a rubber bougie to push the LMAF ETT down through the smooth inner lining of the LMAF, and a standard anesthesia circuit adapter later connected to the end of the LMAF ETT for connection to a breathing circuit. The LMAF is used for urgent or emergent difficult intubation situations and for cannot-ventilate/cannot-intubate situations. Sizing for the LMAF is identical as for other types of LMAs. The proper-sized LMAF is selected according to a patient's weight and by assessing the width of the throat. Once the LMAF is deflated and lubricated with a water-soluble lubricant, it is inserted into the mouth and seated into the superior glottis. The

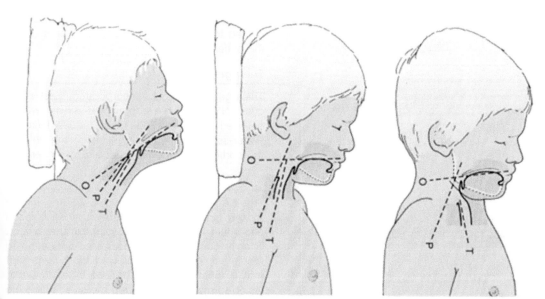

Fig. 18. Correct positioning for ventilation and tracheal intubation. (*From* Fiadjoe JE, Litman RS, Serber JF, et al. The pediatric airway. In: Cote CJ, Lerman J, Anderson BJ, editors. A practice of anesthesia for infants and children. 6th ed. Philadelphia, PA: Elsevier; 2019. p. 297–339; with permission.)

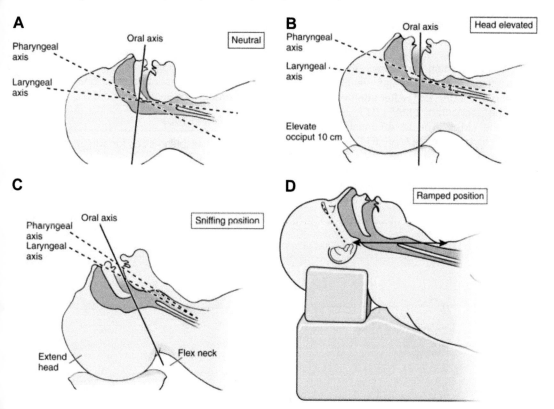

Fig. 19. Head positioning for tracheal intubation. (*A*) Neutral position. (*B*) Head elevated. (*C*) Sniffing position with a flexed neck and extended head. Note that flexing the neck while extending the head lines up the various axes and allows direct laryngoscopy. (*D*) Morbidly obese patients are best intubated in a ramped position with elevation of the upper part of the back, neck, and head; the ideal position aligns the external auditory canal and the sternum. (*From* Reardon RF, McGill JW, Clinton JE. Tracheal intubation. In: Roberts JR, Custalow CB, Thomsen TW, editors. Roberts & Hedges' clinical procedures in emergency medicine. Philadelphia: Saunders; 2014. p. 62–106.e5; with permission.)

the tube and the anesthesia circuit or BVM is connected to deliver positive ventilation pressure to the patient.

The i-gel

The i-gel (Intersurgical Incorporated, East Syracuse, NY) is a rigid supraglottic airway with a gel-filled mask that does not require inflation. Water-soluble lubricant is place on the anterior top portion of the device to facilitate its insertion.

King Airway

The KA is another type of supraglottic airway loosely similar to a combitube. The KA is sized according to the kilogram weight of the patient. The KA consists of a standardized connector to the anesthesia circuit followed by a large cuff that is inflated once the device is fully seated, which forms a seal between the soft palate, the tonsillar pillars, and the posterior portion of the tongue. Progressing downward past the large cuff, the tube portion of the KA contains a large Murphy eye and multiple holes for the delivery of gases toward the glottis. Past the tube portion of the KA is another small cone-shaped balloon, which inflates simultaneously when the large cuff is inflated. This portion is designed to extend into the inlet of the esophagus to prevent reflux of some amount of gastric contents.

Endotracheal Tube

ETTs are available in sizes for adults and children. A standard adult ETT consists of a standardized connector to an anesthesia circuit, the ETT, followed by a low-pressure/high-volume cuff that is inserted just past the vocal cords. The inflated

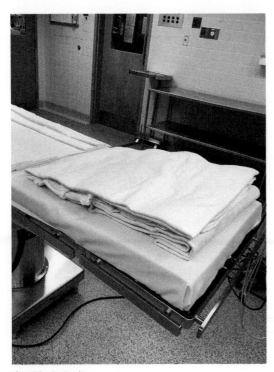

Fig. 20. Ramping.

LMAF mask portion contains an epiglottis retractor flap, which facilitates ventilation and insertion of the LMAF ETT. After attempting ventilation, the lubricated LMAF ETT is inserted through the LMAF. The LMAF mask portion is angulated to guide the LMAF ETT directly into the glottis. The rubber bougie is used to hold the LMAF ETT in place while the LMAF is extracted from the superior glottis. The anesthesia circuit LMAF ETT adapter is inserted onto

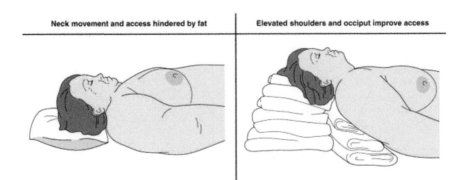

Fig. 21. Positioning the obese patient. Correct positioning is important to optimize the view during laryngoscopy. Flexion of the lower cervical spine brings the trachea in line with the pharynx, and extension at the atlantooccipital joint aligns the trachea with the oral cavity. With the obese patient in the supine position, neck movement and access with a laryngoscope are hindered by fat. When the patient is repositioned with the shoulders elevated and the occiput further elevated so that the head assumes a sniffing position, access to the airway is facilitated. (*From* Wiener-Kronish JP, Shimabukuro DW. Airway management. In: Albert RK, Spiro SG, Jett JR, editors. Clinical respiratory medicine. 3rd edition. Philadelphia: Mosby; 2008. p. 274; with permission.)

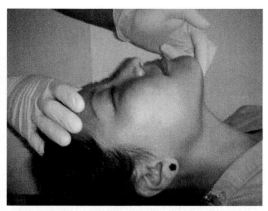

Fig. 22. Airway maintenance using head tilt–chin lift maneuver. (*From* Malamed SF. Intravenous sedation: complications. In: Sedation. St Louis (MO): Elsevier; 2018. p. 380–98; with permission.)

ETT cuff provides an efficient seal against aspiration of gastric contents. An ETT for children less than 8 years of age consists of only standard connector to the anesthesia circuit and a straight plastic tube with no cuff or Murphy eye.

The reinforced adult nonkinking Oral Endotracheal Tube is designed for bending of the tube away from the oral surgical site without kinking of the lumen. The nonkinking tube consists of a flexible plastic with wire reinforcement to hold the lumen open.

Endotracheal Tube Stylet

This plastic-coated malleable metal rod, the ETT stylet, provides correct shape and rigidity to the ETT to help guide the ETT into the glottis.

Eschmann Stylet

This elongated plastic flexible stylette, the Eschmann Stylet (ES), has a bend or coudé tip at its end to aid in the guidance of the stylet into the glottis during a difficult airway situation. The ES is inserted during laryngoscopy through the glottic opening and pushed downward toward the carina. The laryngoscope is removed, and an ETT is threaded along the ES and guided down

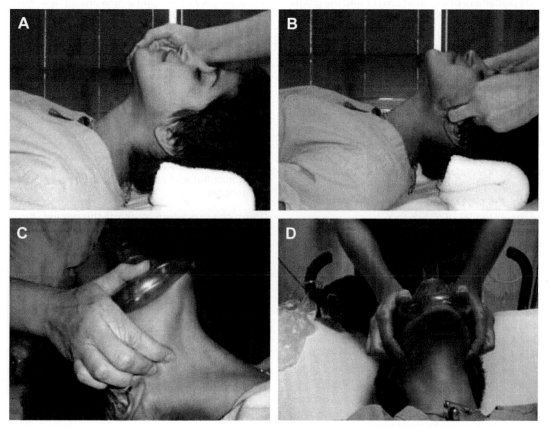

Fig. 23. (*A*) Chin lift into sniffing position. (*B*) Jaw thrust. (*C*) Good mask position with 1 hand. (*D*) Good mask position with 2 hands. (*From* Al-Otaibi Z, Chawla LS. Treatment of medical emergencies. In: Mauro MA, Murphy KPJ, Thomson KR, et al, editors. Image-guided interventions. Philadelphia: Saunders; 2014. p. 54–8.e1; with permission.)

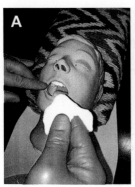 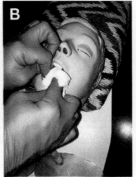 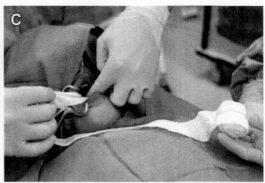

Fig. 24. (*A, B*) Surgical throat pack with a closed system airway. (*C*) Surgical throat pack with an open system airway. (*From* Weddell JA, Jones JE, Emhardt JD. Hospital dental services for children and the use of general anesthesia. In: Dean JA, editor. McDonald and Avery's dentistry for the child and adolescent. St Louis (MO): Elsevier; 2016. p. 328–48; with permission.)

the pathway of the ES through the glottis, while holding the ES securely in position.

Magill Forceps

The Magill Grasping Forceps are available in adult and pediatric sizes. Magill forceps are used to guide placement of the tip of an ETT into the glottis during a nasal intubation and also to precisely and firmly grasp a foreign body for precise removal from the airway.

Laryngeal Tracheal Anesthesia

A laryngeal tracheal anesthesia (LTA) kit consists of a glass vial with 5 mL of 4% plain lidocaine, which is screwed into a long plastic tube with multiple holes around its perimeter near the end of the tube. The LTA is used to anesthetize the glottic inlet during laryngoscopy and prior to intubation for avoidance of the noxious stimulation for patients who cannot tolerate the physiologic stress during purchase of the airway during laryngoscopy.

Airtraq SP

The Airtraq SP is an inexpensive single use disposable video laryngoscope.[31,32] It consists of an antifogging light, a view box, and a blade. The blade allows attachment of the ETT through a channel along its side. The Airtraq is inserted along the midline of the mouth and throat and is then guided toward the vallecula for visualization of the glottic inlet and the vocal cords. The ETT is advanced along the identical path of the blade via the channel and visualized passing through the vocal cords. The Airtraq has been chosen for the American Association of Oral and Maxillofacial Surgeons simulation program because of its ease of use, low cost, and ease of training. There are many other video laryngoscopes available on the market, such as the C-MAC (Karl Storz, Endoscopy-America Inc., El Segundo, CA), the McGRATH laryngoscope (Medtronic, MN), the GlideScope, and the King Vision Video Laryngoscope.

AIRWAY EMERGENCIES

Adverse events in dental anesthesia are most often related to loss of the airway. Maintenance of the airway and recognition of impending airway embarrassment through careful monitoring of a patient's chest rise, use of precordial stethoscope, and monitoring of end-tidal carbon dioxide and pulse oximetry are keys to patient safety. The oral and maxillofacial surgery difficult airway algorithm is shown in **Box 2**. If an airway challenge

---

Box 2
The American Society of Anesthesiologists oral and maxillofacial surgery difficult airway algorithm

Stop the procedure, pack off the wound, suction the oral pharynx, and confirm sniffing position. Increase fraction of inspired oxygen.

Improved or not improved?

Place an oral or nasopharyngeal airway and attempt BVM, either single-handed or 2-handed technique.

Improved or not improved? Call 911?

Place supraglottic airway[a]—consider LMA unique

Improved or not improved? Call 911?

Place ETT and secure airway. Consider a video laryngoscope. Call 911.

[a] Exceptions to placement of a supraglottic airway may include foreign body, severe aspiration, anaphylaxis, and postobstructive pulmonary edema.

occurs, the clear majority can be managed by effective BVM, with some rare exceptions. A common error is to attempt BVM without an airway. Placement of an airway accomplishes 2 of the 3 tasks of the triple airway maneuver and makes BVM much more predictable. It is vitally important to understand the rapidity with which these steps need to be accomplished in opening an airway and ventilating the patient. The oxygen saturation curve is nonlinear and tissue hypoxemia occurs at Saturation Pulsatile of Oxygen levels of 90% and less. The other strong advice when reviewing this algorithm is to call 911 early when difficulty arises. A common theme in adverse events is waiting too long to call for help. It bears mentioning again that if patient selection has been performed carefully, when an emergency occurs, airway management is more predictable.

Preparation for emergencies other than airway management is beyond the scope of this article. Suffice it to say that careful patient selection, team training for specific roles in patient management, crew resource management principles, use of cognitive aids, and having appropriate drugs and equipment available are all essential to safe management of office based anesthesia. Purchase of an airway manikin can be helpful in training staff and performing mock drills. Regular mock drills are essential for team preparation for possible emergencies.

SUMMARY

Poor outcomes in dental anesthesia are almost always related to primary respiratory events and then secondary cardiovascular collapse. Careful patient selection and exclusion of patients as candidates for office anesthetics are an important foundation for patient safety. Utilization of the screening tools described identifies those patients who are not appropriate candidates for office based anesthesia. Knowledge of various airway adjuncts allows for successful management of the airway in the perioperative period. Lastly, understanding emergency algorithms and having a trained anesthesia team allow for successful management of airway emergencies.

REFERENCES

1. Min JJ, Kim G, Kim E. The diagnostic validity of clinical airway assessments for predicting difficult laryngoscopy using a grey zone approach. J Int Med Res 2016;44:893–904.
2. Wajekar AS, Chellam S, Toal PV. Prediction of ease of laryngoscopy and intubation-role of upper lip bite test, modified mallampati classification, and thyromental distance in various combination. J Family Med Prim Care 2015;4:101–5.
3. Hirmanpour A, Safavi M, Honarmand, et al. The predictive value of the ratio of neck circumference to thyromental distance in comparison with four predictive tests for difficult laryngoscopy in obstetric patients scheduled for caesarean delivery. Adv Biomed Res 2014;3:200.
4. Honarmand A, Safavi M, Ansari N. A comparison of between hyomental distance ratios, ratio of height to thyromental, modified Mallamapati classification test and upper lip bite test in predicting difficult laryngoscopy of patients undergoing general anesthesia. Adv Biomed Res 2014;3:166.
5. Safavi M, Honarmand A, Amoushahi M. Prediction of difficult laryngoscopy: extended mallampati score versus the MMT, ULBT and RHTMD. Adv Biomed Res 2014;28(3):133.
6. Ambesh SP, Singh N, Rao PB, et al. A combination of the modified Mallampati score, thyromental distance, anatomical abnormality, and cervical mobility (M-TAC) predicts difficult laryngoscopy better than Mallampati classification. Acta Anaesthesiol Taiwan 2013;51:58–62.
7. Adamus M, Fritscherova S, Hrabalek L, et al. Mallampati test as a predictor of laryngoscopic view. Biomed Pap Med Fac Univ Palacky Olomouc Czech Repub 2010;154:339–43.
8. Cattano D, Panicucci E, Paolicchi A, et al. Risk factors assessment of the difficult airway: an italian survey of 1956 patients. Anesth Analg 2004;99:1774–9.
9. Iohom G, Ronayne M, Cunningham AJ. Prediction of difficult tracheal intubation. Eur J Anaesthesiol 2003;20:31–6.
10. Mallampati SR. Clinical sign to predict difficult tracheal intubation (hypothesis). Can Anaesth Soc J 1983;30:316–7.
11. Mallampati SR, Gatt SP, Gugino LD, et al. A clinical sign to predict difficult tracheal intubation; a prospective study. Can Anaesth Soc J 1985;32:429–34.
12. Tantri AR, Firdaus R, Salomo ST. Predictors of difficult intubation among Malay patients in Indonesia. Anesth Pain Med 2016;6(2):e34848.
13. Inal MT, Memiş D, Sahin SH, et al. Comparison of different tests to determine difficult intubation in pediatric patients. Rev Bras Anestesiol 2014;64:391–4.
14. Safavi M, Honarmand A, Zare N. A comparison of the ratio of patient's height to thyromental distance with the modified Mallampati and the upper lip bite test in predicting difficult laryngoscopy. Saudi J Anaesth 2011;5:258–63.
15. Ittichaikulthol W, Chanpradub S, Amnoundetchakorn S, et al. Modified Mallampati test and thyromental distance as a predictor of difficult laryngoscopy in Thai patients. J Med Assoc Thai 2010;93:84–9.

16. Bindra A, Prabhakar H, Singh GP, et al. Is the modified Mallampati test performed in supine position a reliable predictor of difficult tracheal intubation? J Anesth 2010;24(3):482–5.

17. Mashour GA, Sandberg WS. Craniocervical extension improves the specificity and predictive value of the Mallampati airway evaluation. Anesth Analg 2006;103:1256–9.

18. Ezri T, Warters RD, Szmuk P, et al. The incidence of class "zero" airway and the impact of Mallampati score, age, sex, and body mass index on prediction of laryngoscopy grade. Anesth Analg 2001;93:1073–5.

19. Samsoon GL, Young JR. Difficult tracheal intubation: a retrospective study. Anaesthesia 1987;42:487–90.

20. Colak A, Yilmaz A, Sut N, et al. Investigation of the availability of tongue movements in Mallampati classification. Saudi Med J 2011;32:607–11.

21. Voyagis GS, Kyriakis KP, Dimitriou V, et al. Value of oropharyngeal Mallampati classification in predicting difficult laryngoscopy among obese patients. Eur J Anaesthesiol 1998;15:330–4.

22. Krobbuaban B, Diregpoke S, Kumkeaw S, et al. The predictive value of the height ratio and thyromental distance: four predictive tests for difficult laryngoscopy. Anesth Analg 2005;101:1542–5.

23. Merah NA, Wong DT, Foulkes-Crabbe DJ, et al. Modified Mallampati test, thyromental distance and inter-incisor gap are the best predictors of difficult laryngoscopy in West Africans. Can J Anaesth 2005;52:291–6.

24. Blumenreich GA. Res ipsa loquitur: dental damage during anesthesia. AANA J 1997;65:33–6.

25. Posner K. Closed claim project shows safety evolution. Available at: http://www.apsf.org/newsletters/html/2001/fall/02closedclaims.htm. Accessed March 22, 2017.

26. MacRae M. Closed claims studies in anesthesia: a literature review and implications for practice. AANA J 2007;75:267–75.

27. Schwartz AJ. Insertion of a folded laryngeal mask airway around a palatal torus. AANA J 2005;73:211–6.

28. Sharma D, Prabhakar H, Bithal PK, et al. Predicting difficult laryngoscopy in acromegaly: a comparison of upper lip bite test with modified Mallampati classification. J Neurosurg Anesthesiol 2010;22:138–43.

29. Khan ZH, Kashfi A, Ebrahimkhani E. A comparison of the upper lip bite test (a simple new technique) with modified Mallampati classification in predicting difficulty in endotracheal intubation: a prospective blinded study. Anesth Analg 2003;96:595–9.

30. Schwartz AJ. Dislocation of the mandible: a case report. AANA J 2000;68:507–13.

31. Ertürk T, Deniz S, Şimşek F, et al. Comparison of the Macintosh and Airtraq laryngoscopes in endotracheal intubation success. Turk J Anaesthesiol Reanim 2015;43:181–7.

32. Apfelbaum JL, Hagberg CA, Caplan RA, et al. Practice guidelines for management of the difficult airway: an updated report by the American Society of Anesthesiologists Task Force on Management of the Difficult Airway. Anesthesiology 2013;118:251–70.

APPENDIX 1: SAMPLE OF A SYSTEMS-BASED MEDICAL HISTORY

Anesthesia Health History

1. Patient Information

Today's date_____ Age_____ Birth date_____ Weight_____ Height_____ Sex M or F

Name_____ Home Phone_____

      Last   First   Middle Init.   Cell Phone_____

Home Address_____ City_____ State_____ Zip Code_____

Employer_____ Work Phone_____

Work Address_____ City_____ State_____ Zip Code_____

Spouse / Parent(s) / Guardian(s) Name(s)_____

Address_____ City_____ State_____ Home Phone_____

Person to contact in case of **emergency**_____ Phone_____

Address_____ City_____ State_____ Home Phone_____

---

2. Patient Medical History

Physician Name_____ Office Phone_____

Date of Last Exam_____ Reason for last visit_____

		Yes	No			Yes	No
1.	Are you under the care of a physician?	☐	☐	7.			
2.	Have you ever been hospitalized for any surgical operation or serious illness?	☐	☐		Are you allergic to or have you had any reaction to the following?		
					Local Anesthetics	☐	☐
3.	If yes, describe_____				Penicillin or any antibiotics	☐	☐
					Sulfa drugs	☐	☐
4.	Do you use tobacco?	☐	☐		Aspirin	☐	☐
5.	Do you wear contact lenses?	☐	☐		Codeine	☐	☐
					Other_____		
6.	Are you taking any medications, non-prescription medications, herbal medicines, vitamins?	☐	☐				

Please list_____

8. Do you now, or have you had any of the following?

Respiratory/Lungs   Yes   No

	Yes	No
Recent Cold	☐	☐
Pneumonia / Cough /Flu	☐	☐
Asthma/Bronchitis	☐	☐
Emphysema	☐	☐
Short of Breath	☐	☐
Easily Winded	☐	☐
Tuberculosis	☐	☐

Musculoskeletal

	Yes	No
Arthritis/Back or Hip Problem	☐	☐
Joint replacement/Implant	☐	☐
Muscle weakness/Paralysis	☐	☐
Numbness/Tingling	☐	☐

Neurological

	Yes	No
Fainting	☐	☐
Epilepsy/Convulsions/Seizures	☐	☐
Psychiatric treatment/Nervous	☐	☐
Stroke/Transient ischemic attac	☐	☐

Cardiovascular   Yes   No

	Yes	No
Mitral valve prolapse	☐	☐
Rheumatic fever	☐	☐
High/ Low Blood pressure	☐	☐
Abnormal Rhythm	☐	☐
Peripheral Vascular Disease	☐	☐
Blood clots	☐	☐
Leukemia or anemia	☐	☐
Blood transfusion	☐	☐
Bleeding difficulty	☐	☐
Heart disease	☐	☐
Congestive **Heart** Failure	☐	☐
Swollen ankles	☐	☐
Cardiac Pacemaker/AICD	☐	☐
Heart murmur	☐	☐
Congenital heart lesions	☐	☐
Heart Attack	☐	☐
Angina	☐	☐
Chest Pain	☐	☐
Cardiac Stent	☐	☐

Liver/Kidneys   Yes   No

	Yes	No
Kidney diseases	☐	☐
Hepatitis/Jaundice	☐	☐
Liver Disease	☐	☐

Other

	Yes	No
Diabetes	☐	☐
AIDS HIV STD	☐	☐
Frequently tired	☐	☐
Thyroid disease	☐	☐
Cancer	☐	☐
Stomach trouble/Nausea	☐	☐
Hiatal hernia	☐	☐
Gastric reflux	☐	☐
Hay fever/Seasonal allergy	☐	☐
Radiation Therapy	☐	☐
Glaucoma	☐	☐
Recent weight gain loss	☐	☐
Cold Sores	☐	☐

9. *Women only:*

	Yes	No
a) Are you pregnant?	☐	☐
b) Do you think you may be pregnant?	☐	☐
c) Are you nursing?	☐	☐
d) Are you taking Birth Control Pills?	☐	☐

Are you _now using_ or have you _ever used_ drugs such as:

Cocaine, heroine, methamphetamine, marijuana or others? Yes ☐ No ☐

_____   _____

Patient Signature   **Date**

_____   _____

Doctor Signature /Anesthesia Provider Signature   **Date**

Updated_____

Anesthetic Pump Techniques Versus the Intermittent Bolus
What the Oral Surgeon Needs to Know

Richard C. Robert, DDS, MS*, Chirag M. Patel, DMD, MD

KEYWORDS

- Rapid redistribution • GABAA receptor • Context-sensitive half-time • Infusion pump
- Hybrid analog-digital • Smart technology

KEY POINTS

- Most of the agents currently in use for office-based anesthesia have rapid onset and offset and exert their effects through binding to receptor sites on ligand-activated ion channels in the central nervous system.
- To sustain a "smooth" anesthetic effect, anesthetic receptor sites require a steady source of agent molecules from the bloodstream.
- Although the incremental bolus approach to anesthetic delivery has served oral and maxillofacial surgeons well for decades, infusion pumps may offer advantages that should be considered.
- Although no longer in production, the hybrid analog-digital infusion pump introduced by Bard and Baxter over two decades ago continues to be popular in hospitals, outpatient surgery centers, and oral and maxillofacial surgeons' offices.
- New digital infusion pumps have "smart technology" that enables verification of the syringe, confirmation of drug dosing, and computer interfacing.

INTRODUCTION AND HISTORY

Since the seminal work of Wells and Morton in the 1840s,[1] the specialty of oral and maxillofacial surgery has been on a quest to find the ideal anesthetic for office-based oral and maxillofacial surgery. This quest has progressed from nitrous oxide to a number of intravenous agents including ultrashort-acting barbiturates, benzodiazepines, opioids, the dissociative anesthetic ketamine, and most recently the alkylated phenol propofol.[2] The quest of our specialty somewhat parallels that seen in anesthesia for ambulatory surgery. By the end of the previous century, far more procedures were performed on an ambulatory basis as opposed to protracted hospitalizations. This transition was largely fueled by the availability of such agents as propofol, ketamine, and remifentanil, which provided more rapid recovery with less likelihood of postoperative nausea and vomiting or respiratory depression. For delivery of these agents, oral and maxillofacial surgeons (OMSs) have relied on small, incremental boluses to sustain the anesthetic effect. However, many anesthesiologists have found that infusion pumps can provide a smoother anesthetic course, and now most prefer this approach.[3] The reasons that anesthesiologists overcame their initial reluctance to use infusion pumps and the potential advantages for OMSs is explored.

No disclosures regarding financial or commercial interests.

Department of Oral and Maxillofacial Surgery, University of California at San Francisco School of Dentistry, Box 0440, 533 Parnassus Avenue, UB 10, San Francisco, CA 94143, USA

* Corresponding author.

E-mail address: rcr2400@aol.com

Oral Maxillofacial Surg Clin N Am 30 (2018) 227–237
https://doi.org/10.1016/j.coms.2018.02.001
1042-3699/18/

The Nature of Current Anesthetic Agents Used for Office-Based Anesthesia

Propofol[4] and other currently popular agents such as ketamine and remifentanil[5] owe that popularity to their rapid onset and short duration. It has been found that the agents with these characteristics are often associated with less postoperative headache, nausea, and vomiting as compared with their predecessors such as methohexital[6] and fentanyl.[7] In addition, some of these agents can be used in combination to capitalize on the desirable effects of both. For example, Mortero and colleagues[8] found that the coadministration of low-dose ketamine attenuates propofol-induced hypoventilation and may lead to earlier return of cognition postoperatively as well. As the advantages of the newer agents became more widely appreciated, both anesthesiologists and OMSs began to incorporate them into their practices.

After decades of success with methohexital delivered by an incremental bolus technique, most OMSs adopted the same approach to the delivery of propofol and ketamine. In the meantime, anesthesiologists worked with equipment engineers to develop infusion pumps, which they felt would take better advantage of the pharmacologic attributes of the new agents.[9] Even in the case of medically compromised patients, they found that the latter approach could provide hemodynamic stability as well as simplicity of delivery.[10] Like OMSs, they had originally used an incremental bolus approach, but they ultimately found that infusion pumps could better serve their needs. They concluded that the optimal delivery of the new agents would be best accomplished with the steady infusion provided by an infusion pump.[11] This steady infusion could then also make it possible for the anesthesiologist to use intravenous agents to maintain a continuous level of anesthesia comparable with that which heretofore had only been possible with halogenated inhalation agents. The next section explores the rationale for anesthesiologist adoption of infusion pumps as their preferred means of delivery for intravenous anesthesia.

The Rationale for the Use of Infusion Pumps

The rationale for anesthesiologists' adopting infusion pumps as their primary mode of delivery of intravenous (IV) anesthetic agents is based on studies in the 1980s and 1990s on the dissipation of drug effect.[12] It was determined that the decrease in the plasma concentration of lipophilic anesthetic drugs after administration is due more to redistribution than actual metabolism or elimination. After passage through the blood–brain barrier, these IV anesthetic molecules bind to their respective receptor sites on ligand-activated ion channels in the central nervous system, but only briefly. They then return to central circulation and are rapidly distributed to the other tissues of the body.[13] For the activity of these agents to be continued for the duration of the anesthetic, new anesthetic molecules must be constantly available from the central circulation to again bind with the receptor site. **Fig. 1** illustrates this dynamic interaction between propofol and the gamma-amino butyric acid-A receptor.[14]

Once the anesthetic molecules have left the receptor sites, they are not distributed to all of the body's tissues equally, largely owing to differences in local blood flow. Physiologists have empirically divided the tissues into 3 groups or "compartments" based on vascularity. The first of these is the "vessel-rich group," consisting of the brain, heart, kidneys, and other highly vascularized tissues. The second or "intermediate group" consists of less well-perfused tissues such as muscle and skin. The third or "vessel-poor" compartment includes poorly perfused tissues such as bone and fat. After the infusion has been discontinued, the anesthetic molecules return from the latter compartments and reenter the central circulation. They are transported to the liver, where they are biotransformed and then excreted through the kidneys. It should be pointed out that the compartments are not anatomic entities, but theoretic ones based on mathematical calculations.

As these lipophilic anesthetic molecules pass through the central and peripheral compartments, the effect site requires new anesthetic molecules if the anesthetic effect is to be maintained. Then, once the infusion has been discontinued, there is a rapid decrease in the serum concentration depending on the drug under consideration. The parameter that most accurately captures this dynamic relationship is the context-sensitive half-time, that is, the time required for a 50% reduction in serum concentration after discontinuation of the infusion.[15] In **Fig. 2**, the plots for propofol and ketamine are compared with those of their predecessors sodium thiopental and methohexital. The low, relatively flat plots of propofol and ketamine are consistent with their clinical attribute of being associated with earlier discharge times as compared with many other agents. The plot for remifentanil is even lower and flatter than those of propofol and ketamine. This shape is a reflection of its rapid metabolism by esterases throughout the body, as opposed to hepatic biotransformation.[16]

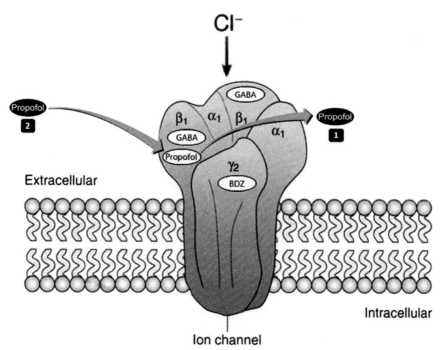

Fig. 1. The gamma-amino butyric acid-A (GABA) receptor. As the bond between the propofol receptor site and propofol molecule 1 is broken and it returns to the central circulation (redistribution), the constant infusion transports in propofol molecule 2 to sustain the opening of the chloride channel. BDZ, benzodiazepine. (*Modified from* Reves JG, Glass PSA, Lubarsky DA, et al. Intravenous nonopioid anesthetics. In: Miller RD, editor. Miller's anesthesia. 6th edition. New York: Elsevier/Churchill Livingstone; 2005. p. 337; with permission.)

To ensure a consistently "smooth" anesthetic course the slow, unceasing replenishing of agents to their respective receptors sites requires a

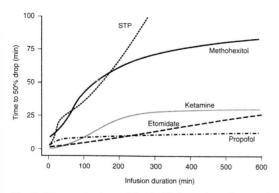

Fig. 2. The context sensitive half-time plot of several intravenous anesthetic agents. Note the low, flat plot for propofol, which correlates closely with rapid recovery and readiness for discharge. (*Adapted from* Loose E, Egan TD. Short-acting intravenous anesthetics. In: Springman S, editor. Ambulatory anesthesia: the requisites in anesthesiology. 1st edition. Philadelphia: Mosby; 2006. p. 38; with permission; and Egan TD. Pharmacokinetics and rational intravenous drug selection and administration in anesthesia. In: Lake CI, Rice I, Sperry RJ, editors. Advances in anesthesia. vol. 12. St Louis (MO): Mosby; 1995; with permission.)

constant infusion. Although an intermittent or incremental bolus approach can simulate this action to a limited extent, it cannot compare with the unwaveringly steady delivery provided by an infusion pump. Consequently, anesthesiologists have tended to favor IV anesthetic delivery via infusion pumps as opposed to an incremental bolus approach.[17]

Interestingly, since the 1990s studies published in primary OMS journals, like those in anesthesia journals, have pointed to the benefits of infusion pump delivery in office-based OMS surgery. For instance, in 1995 Candelaria and Smith[18] commented that, "An infusion pump enables achievement of a sustained sedative-hypnotic effect without oscillations between peak and trough levels in the blood and brain, producing varying levels of anesthetic depths." Then, in 1998, Bennett and colleagues[19] concluded that, "The continuous infusion of propofol was associated with an anesthesia level that was statistically superior in both minimizing patient movement and providing a more optimal overall quality of anesthesia." Although each year there has been a slow increase in the percentage of OMS offices using pumps, they remain in the distinct minority. This finding raises the question as to what

OMSs need to know for them to become more comfortable with the idea of using an infusion pump for delivery of their anesthetics. In this article, we attempt to answer these questions.

Why Are Oral and Maxillofacial Surgeons Not Routinely Using Infusion Pumps?

The major objections that OMSs have posed to the use of infusion pumps are similar to those originally posed by anesthesiologists.[20] These objections have been explored thoroughly in the anesthesia literature and no evidence was found to support them.[17] Many of the objections involve expense, such as the cost of the pump. However, in the average OMS office performing hundreds of anesthetics per year, the initial outlay is rapidly recouped within a year or two. The devices are solidly constructed with the finest of engineering and electronic input. Many pumps in current use have been in service for decades with no signs of deterioration. Consequently, the cost per patient over that extended period of time is only about $0.25. The syringes for drug administration are identical to those required for the incremental bolus technique such that there is no difference in cost on that basis. The connection between the pump and the IV line is an inexpensive IV extension costing approximately $0.75. Thus, the total difference in cost between using an infusion pump versus the incremental bolus technique is probably only about $1 per patient.

Another concern is the perceived relinquishing of anesthetic care of the patient to a machine. As for safety, it has been amply demonstrated in the literature that the least safe method of medication administration is via bolus by an unmonitored provider. Such errors have been attributed to distraction, inattention, and failure to carefully read drug vial labels.[21] The newer infusion pumps with "smart technology" require verification of settings before drug delivery and even verify the brand and size of the syringe that has been placed in the pump. Once the settings have been entered by the first provider, they can be rechecked by a second observer, providing another element of safety.[22]

Another concern is the erroneous perception that extensive extra time is required for setting up the pump before the case. Because syringes need to be loaded and attached to the IV line for both pump and for incremental bolus delivery, these times are similar. If the pump is kept in the operative suite on its mounting bracket, essentially the only extra time required during set up is entering the pump settings, which takes only 20 to 30 seconds.

TYPES OF PUMPS

Automatic syringe pumps are most frequently types of pumps used in anesthesia. They consist of a screw-drive mechanism controlled by a servo motor. Operation of these infusion pumps is actually quite simple in comparison with other devices commonly in use in OMS offices such as anesthetic monitors and cone beam computed tomography (CBCT) machines. Syringe pumps can be divided into 2 major types, either hybrid analog/digital or full digital. In the sections that follow, we examine the operation of each of these 2 types of pumps.

Hybrid Analog/Digital Such as the Baxter Infuse OR

Although no longer in production, this hybrid analog-digital infusion pump introduced by Bard and Baxter (Baxter Healthcare Corporation, Deerfield, IL) more than 2 decades ago continues to be popular in hospitals, outpatient surgery centers, and OMS offices (**Fig. 3**A). These pumps can still be found on the market as refurbished units and tend to command a purchase price comparable with the newer digital pumps described herein. The development of this pump by Bard (and subsequently sold to Baxter) was a pivotal event in surgical health care. In the latter decades of the 20th century, ambulatory surgery overtook overnight hospital surgery as the primary mode for the delivery of surgical care. Technological advances reduced surgical morbidity significantly, and it became possible for patients to have "day-stay" procedures. In addition, medicinal chemists developed such agents as propofol and alfentanil, which enhanced readiness for discharge consistent with the day-study model. Anesthesiologists felt that these agents would be best delivered by an infusion pump. However, up until the 1980s, infusion pumps were large, bulky, and not user friendly. Consequently, when Baxter began to market a new type of pump, the simple syringe pump, anesthesiologists were prompt to adopt them.

The Baxter pump was imaginatively innovative and remarkably intuitive. It relied on simple syringes for delivery, not unlike the delivery of anesthetic agents with syringes performed by anesthesiologists on an everyday basis. Rather than relying on the anesthesiologist' thumb to depress the plunger, the pump mechanism did so based on settings entered by the operator with dials on the face of the pump. The big difference was that the slow, consistent depression of the plunger during maintenance with the infusion pump provided a steady supply of anesthetic molecules to receptors, rather than the intermittent

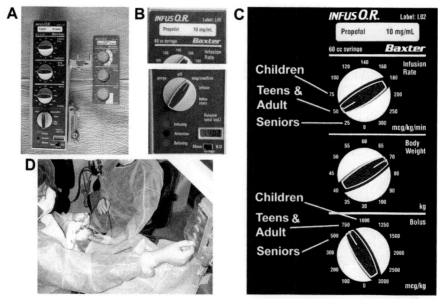

Fig. 3. (*A*) Baxter Infuse OR infusion pump with the adult propofol face plate mounted and a pediatric propofol face plate on the right for comparison. (*B*) Top portion of the adult propofol face plate showing the label on the top right that should match on the LCD display when the Mode dial is turned to "Stop/confirm." (*C*) Adult propofol face plate showing suggested infusion rates and bolus amounts for different age groups. (*D*) Photo depicting ease of use of the Baxter Infuse OR pump intraoperatively.

one provided by handheld syringes. Setting up the pump was simple and merely required entering the desired settings on the dials on the pump face, which only took a few seconds. Thus, the pump could be programmed quite easily with dosing virtually identical to that which the anesthesiologists had been delivering manually for years.

The Baxter pump has specific interchangeable electromagnetic templates for each drug and patient type (adult vs pediatric; see **Fig. 3**A). The pump is automatically programmed for use with a particular drug based on the face plate chosen. On the face of the Baxter pump there are 4 programming dials that are used to adjust various parameters determined by the specific face plate used (see **Fig. 3**A). These dials provide adjustment of the infusion rate, patient weight, bolus size, and the lower dial activates the pump.

The continued popularity of the Baxter pump is based on a quick setup time and ease of operation. Its disadvantages include that (1) there is no "confirmation" when changes are made, (2) the pump is designed for use with 60-mL syringes only, (3) the bolus rate is fixed and cannot be changed (a minor disadvantage), and (4) there is no interface to pair with a computer.

Baxter pump users have not been deterred by what they perceive as minor disadvantages of the pump, and many of these pumps have been in regular use for 15 years or longer in hospitals,

outpatient surgery centers, and OMS offices. Refurbishing is relatively inexpensive and many of the older units have seen a second life.

Newer Digital Pumps with "Smart Technology"

The Atlanta Biomedical Corporation (Suwanee, GA) Model 4100 will be used as an example of a typical digital pump. Rather than dials, these units have a digital keypad that is used for programming and operation (**Fig. 4**A). There is digital memory for storing settings for an extensive library of drugs. Some additional advantages include the following. (1) Smaller syringes can be used, which provide greater accuracy for long infusions at low rates.[23] (2) They incorporate a confirmation mode whenever a setting is changed, thereby ensuring an additional layer of safety. This mode protects the operator from using pump settings from the previous case for the current one. (3) Unlike the Baxter Infuse OR pump, they have the ability to interface with a computer for automatic transfer of data. (4) An additional advantage of digital pumps is the ability to control the rate of delivery of a bolus. Although these devices are slightly less "user friendly" than the Baxter pump, there is still a relatively short learning curve. For those who have previous experience with the Baxter pump, it is quite easy to convert the settings from one pump to the other.

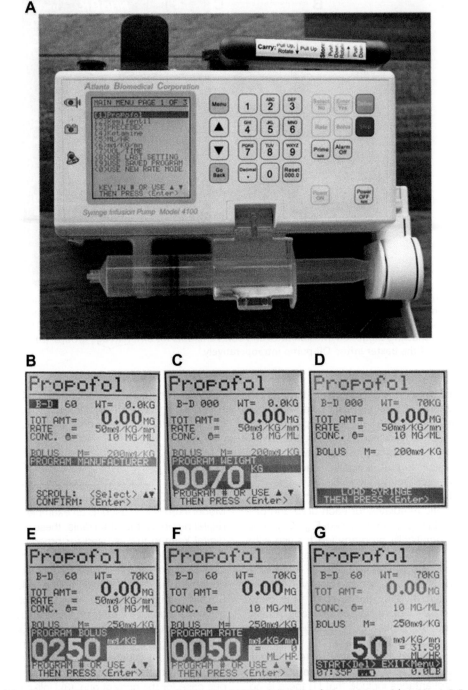

Fig. 4. (*A*) Atlanta BioMedical Corporation (Suwanee, GA) Model 4100 infusion pump with a 60-mL B-D syringe. (*B–G*) Screenshots of the LCD screen depicting steps involved in setting up the pump for a propofol infusion as described in the text.

OPERATION
Office-Based Anesthesia with Infusion Pumps

Preanesthestic and preinduction medications
As has been noted with the incremental bolus technique, preanesthetic and preinduction

medications tend to enhance the overall quality of a pump delivered anesthetic. There are 2 orally administered agents that have been used to good effect. One of these is clonidine, an alpha-2 agonist, that, when given before the primary anesthetic, helps to counteract adrenergic and hypothalamopituitary stress response.[24] It also reduces secretions and has antiemetic and analgesic properties. A second very popular preinduction medication is midazolam, which provides anxiolysis and enhances amnesia early in the course of the anesthetic to avoid recall of unpleasant events, such as the stinging from propofol.[25] Also quite helpful is the administration of a 1.5- to 2.0-mg "test dose" of propofol along with the other preinduction medications. The response of the patient to this test dose helps to guide the operator in determining the dose of the preinduction bolus as discussed elsewhere in this article.

Patient characteristics

There are several patient characteristics that should be taken into account, regardless of whether the method of delivery is via the incremental bolus technique or an infusion pump. These characteristics include the following.

1. Weight – Generally, the greater the weight, the more drug the patient will require. However, for obese and morbidly obese patients, the induction bolus should be determined by lean body mass rather than total body weight.
2. Gender – It has been well-documented in the anesthesia literature that a higher induction dose and infusion rate is required for women as opposed to men.[26]
3. Age – Extremes of age require medication adjustment. Geriatric patients have a smaller volume of distribution, which requires reduced dosages. On the opposite end of the age spectrum, pediatric patients have a large volume of distribution, which requires increased induction and maintenance dosages.
4. Habitus and possible obstructive sleep apnea – In the event of an airway emergency, the obese and morbidly obese patient, especially those with obstructive sleep apnea, pose formidable challenges. Consequently, the induction bolus should be based on lean body mass rather than total body weight.
5. Medical compromise – Middle-aged and older, frail patients tend to have diminished cardiovascular and pulmonary reserve, and should receive decreased doses of induction and maintenance medications.

When programming either of these pumps, there are 9 parameters that must be taken into account. Once set, most of these parameters are constant for a wide variety of cases, and only 3 need to be routinely customized for the individual patient. The 9 parameters are:

1. Syringe type – brand and size;
2. Drug name;
3. Dosing mode – for example, micrograms per kilogram per minute;
4. Drug concentration;
5. Patient weight – care must be taken to enter the weight in the correct units (kilograms);
6. Infusion rate;
7. Bolus rate – The rate is constant for the Baxter pump and it is 360 mL/h. Four different bolus rates (normal, low, mid, and high) are available with the Atlanta Biomedical Corporation pump;
8. Bolus dose; and
9. Occlusion level.

The 3 parameters that must be customized for each patient include patient weight, infusion rate, and bolus dose. Although the operator also makes adjustments of these parameters when the incremental bolus technique is used, the adjustments tend to be more exact when one uses an infusion pump.

Setting the Bolus

Giving an appropriate induction bolus is critical to the overall success of the anesthetic, and this is another feature in which the infusion pump excels. The slow, smooth delivery of the bolus by the pump promotes hemodynamic stability. Rapid, unevenly delivered boluses given with handheld syringes are prone to enhance the hypotensive and respiratory depressant effects of propofol. The size of the bolus is in large part determined by the anticipated volume of distribution of the given patient and modified by the patient's response to a 1.5- to 2.0-mL test dose given along with the preinduction medications. The principal author's recommended bolus and maintenance infusion dosages for the Baxter pump are illustrated in **Fig. 3**A. These dosages are based on the experience of delivering intravenous anesthetics to several thousand patients. They are consistent with dosages published in the anesthesia literature for outpatient surgery using monitored anesthesia care.

It should be noted that the bolus doses for older patients are markedly reduced. This adjustment is in large part owing to the sensitivity of elderly patients to the hypotensive and respiratory depressive effects of propofol as discussed. For patients over the age of 60, the dosages are reduced further as follow: for patients in their 70s, the dose is reduced to 300 µg/kg, for those in their 80s to 200 µg/kg, and for those in their 90s to 100 µg/kg.

For digital pumps, it is helpful to set up the bolus dose as one-third of the total bolus planned. **Table 1** gives suggested bolus and infusion

Table 1
Dosing guidelines

Teens/Adults	Pediatric	Seniors >65
Induction bolus 250 µg/kg × 2–3	Induction bolus 330 µg/kg × 3	Induction bolus 60's →150 µg/kg × 3 70's →150 µg/kg × 2 80's →150 µg/kg × 1
Infusion rate 50–75 µg/kg/min	Infusion rate 75–100 µg/kg/min	Infusion rate 25 µg/kg/min

dosages for various categories of patients. These doses are based on those previously established for the Baxter Infuse OR pump. For instance, in **Table 1** the induction bolus amount listed for teens and adults is 250 µg/kg which is one-third of the induction bolus of 750 µg/kg recommended for the Baxter pump. In the case of the digital pump, the bolus button is depressed 3 times in succession to give the total bolus dose of 750 µg/kg. When the initial test dose discussed demonstrates that the patient is very sensitive to propofol, 1 or 2 of the 250 µg/kg doses can be administered rather

than the full 3 doses. In addition, it should be noted that the induction boluses listed for seniors in the third column of the table reflect the same decreases with age discussed for the Baxter pump.

Intraoperative Pump Operation

During the maintenance phase of the anesthetic, the infusion rate can be adjusted to increase or decrease the amount of drug delivered. Boluses can also be administered intraoperatively in response to surgical stress with the turn of a dial or push of a button. If the propofol in the original syringe runs out, the syringe can be refilled with the use of a 3-way stopcock. A 20-mL syringe can be connected to the side port of the 3-way stopcock for refilling the main pump syringe.

What follows is a detailed description of how to set up both of theses pumps for infusing propofol using a 60-mL BD syringe.

SETUP AND OPERATION OF THE BAXTER PUMP

As pointed out previously, the intuitive design of the Baxter pump makes it possible for the anesthetist to use it in a manner quite similar to that which is used with the incremental bolus technique. **Table 2** provides a side-by-side comparison of the steps in delivering an anesthetic with

Table 2
Comparison of an incremental bolus with a Baxter infusion pump

	Step	Incremental Bolus Technique	Baxter Infuse OR Pump
1	Set up	Assemble syringe, propofol and connecting tubing.	Assemble syringe, propofol and connecting tubing, confirm propofol plate and the B-D syringe (see **Fig. 3**B)
2	Obtain the patient's weight, convert it to kilograms and prepare for delivering the anesthetic.	Once it has been calculated, record the weight in kilograms for use in calculating the bolus amount and incremental boluses for anesthetic maintenance	Once it has been calculated, the weight in kilograms is entered with the "Body Weight" dial on the face of the pump (see **Fig. 3**C)
3	Determine the bolus amount and infusion maintenance dose	Using the patient's weight in kilograms calculate the number of milliliters of propofol for the bolus (∼5.0 mL) and the incremental boluses (∼2 mL q5min)	Turn the "Bolus" dial to 750 µg/kg and the "Infusion Rate" dial to 50 µg/kg/min (see **Fig. 3**C)
4	Deliver the bolus	Depress the plunger 5 mL	Turn the bottom dial to deliver the bolus
5	Maintain the infusion	Deliver incremental boluses of ∼2 mL q5min	No action required – after delivering the bolus the pump delivers the maintenance infusion of 50 µg/kg/min

each technique. In our example, the patient weighs 70 kg and will be receiving an initial bolus dose of 75 µg/kg followed by an infusion rate of 50 µg/kg/min. When one views the table it is apparent that there are 5 simple steps in each technique and that the steps for the Baxter pump merely mimic those of the incremental bolus technique under the direction of the operator who sets the dials.

For entering the weight in kilograms on the pump, pounds are roughly converted to kilograms by dividing the weight by 2. For males, 10% is subtracted to arrive at the weight in kilograms, and the nearest weight selected on the pump. For females, the step of subtracting 10% from the weight divided by 2 is omitted. The 10% difference in the weight entered on the pump results in an approximate 10% higher dosage for a female patient. This practice is consistent with the anesthesia literature, which indicates that women require approximately 10% to 15% higher dosage levels of propofol than do males.

Fig. 3C shows the suggested propofol boluses for patients of different age groups. The rates shown in **Fig. 3** are based on the differences in the volume of distribution for patients of the various age groups. Thus, patients less than 12 years of age receive a higher dosage, whereas patients over the age of 60 receive a smaller dose, as previously described. If subsequent boluses are required during the procedure, the bolus amount can be adjusted as needed. **Fig. 3**C also demonstrates the suggested infusion rates for patients of different age groups. This can be easily titrated with adjustments of the infusion rate as needed during surgery (see **Fig. 3**D).

The infusion can be stopped at any time by returning the mode dial to "stop/confirm." At this point, the LCD display will show the amount of total drug delivered during the case in milliliters. One should avoid turning the dial to the "off" position, which will erase the total drug amount delivered from the memory.

SETUP AND OPERATION OF A DIGITAL PUMP

As discussed, the Atlanta Biomedical Corporation Model 4100 will be used as our example of a typical digital pump (available from Wilburn Medical Inc, Kernersville, NC). The same principles used in entering settings for the Baxter pump apply to these newer digital infusion pumps. However, rather than entering settings with dials, one presses a key or a button. After the first settings are entered during initial pump set up, most are retained as "default" settings. As in the case of the Baxter pump, for most cases the only settings

that must be individualized for the case are the patient weight, the bolus amount, and the maintenance infusion rate. In **Table 3** there is a side-by-side comparison of the operation of the pumps. The steps are very similar for the 2 pumps, with the obvious exception that the entries on the digital pump are made with a keyboard rather than a dial.

As in the case of the Baxter pump, intraoperative adjustments to the infusion rate or bolus can be made by pressing "Rate" or "Bolus," respectively. At the end of the case, the infusion can be stopped by pressing "Stop."

As one can see, the settings on the digital pump are comparable with those entered on the Baxter pump, with the primary difference being that each setting must be confirmed by pressing "Enter." Although this does entail an additional step, it imparts an additional element of safety because the settings are being confirmed, as opposed to merely entered. This additional step does not appreciably increase the setup time for the pump because it only takes approximately 20 to 30 seconds.

In conclusion, as we have seen from the examples, delivering an intravenous anesthetic with a syringe pump is actually quite similar to delivering one with handheld syringes. Obviously, anesthesiologists have been pleased with the transition they made from manual syringes to syringe pumps. The syringe pump is exceedingly intuitive and does not usurp control of the anesthetic from the operator. Rather, it transfers control of the syringe plunger from the operator's thumb to his or her fingers, which turn the dials or touch the keys. The syringe remains in clear sight with its plunger moving precisely as the operator had intended. However, the movement is much "smoother" than that which the operator could have accomplished with his or her thumb.

There is a certain irony in OMSs' reluctance to adopt infusion pumps in their practices. Our specialty has incorporated a number of technologic advancements within recent years. Conventional radiographs have been replaced by digital ones and CBCT plays an ever-increasing role in imaging. Technologically sophisticated monitors similar to those used in hospital operating rooms are used routinely during anesthesia. Three-dimensional printing enables custom reconstruction plates, and computer-generated splints are used in orthognathic surgery and implant dentistry. Yet, for some inexplicable reason, the relatively simple technology of the syringe pump for intravenous anesthetics has not as yet been adopted by the majority of the members of our specialty. It is hoped that the simple comparison between

Table 3
Comparison of the Baxter infusion pump with a digital pump

	Step	Baxter Infuse OR Pump	Digital Pump
1	Set up	Assemble syringe, propofol and connecting tubing, confirm propofol plate and the B-D syringe (see **Fig. 3**B)	Turn on the pump, confirm propofol (see **Fig. 4**A) and confirm B-D syringe by pressing "Enter" (**Fig. 4**B)
2	Obtain the patient's weight, convert it to kilograms and prepare for delivering the anesthetic.	Once it has been calculated, the weight of 70 kg is entered with the "Body Weight" dial on the face of the pump (see **Fig. 3**C)	Enter the patient's weight of 70 kg in the "PROGRAM WEIGHT" box and press "Enter" (**Fig. 4**C)
3	Determine the bolus amount and infusion maintenance dose	Turn the "Bolus" dial to 750 µg/kg and the "Infusion Rate" dial to 50 µg/kg/min (see **Fig. 3**C)	Follow the prompt to "LOAD THE SYRINGE" (**Fig. 4**D), press enter, program the bolus (250) and the rate (50) and press "Enter" after each (**Fig. 4**E, F)
4	Deliver the bolus	Turn the bottom dial to deliver the 750 µg/kg bolus	Start the infusion (**Fig. 4**G) by pressing the green "Deliver" button (see **Fig. 4**A); press the "Bolus" and "Deliver" buttons 3 times (250 µg/kg × 3 = 750 µg/kg)
5	Maintain the infusion	No action required – after delivering the bolus the pump delivers the maintenance infusion of 50 µg/kg/min	No action required – after delivering the bolus the pump delivers the maintenance infusion of 50 µg/kg/min

manual syringe delivery and syringe pumps we have offered will prompt more OMSs to incorporate this exceedingly helpful technology into their practices.

SUMMARY

The most popular agents currently in use for office-based anesthesia are drugs such as propofol, ketamine, and remifentanil, which have the very desirable properties of rapid onset and offset of action and readiness for discharge. The parameter that best reflects this latter attribute of lipophilic anesthetic agents is the context sensitive half-time. The "smoothness" of the anesthetic is enhanced when there is a steady source of agent molecules available from the central circulation for binding to the receptor sites on the neuronal ion channels. Only an infusion pump can reliably provide this type of consistent, unwavering flow of agent molecules. Although this concept has been embraced by anesthesiologists, OMSs have tended to continue to use the incremental bolus technique, which has served them well for many decades. It is hoped that the good success of anesthesiologists and their colleague OMSs who use infusion pumps will prompt more OMSs to use infusion pumps in the future.

To assist surgeons who are considering the adoption of an infusion pump approach, we have demonstrated how these pumps can be used to provide enhanced drug delivery. Operation of the 2 commonly available types of syringe pumps has been described. The first of these is the hybrid analog-digital Baxter Infuse OR pump that is actually no longer in production. However, owing to its popularity as a user-friendly device with demonstrated reliability and simplicity, it continues to be in widespread use in hospital operating rooms, outpatient surgery centers, and OMS offices. Its popularity is mirrored in the continued availability of refurbished units in the marketplace. The second pump discussed is one of the newer digital pumps that have smart technology that enables them to verify the syringe, confirm anesthetic doses, and provide a computer interface. This article has also addressed the concerns of OMSs who have reservations about the adoption of infusion pumps for the delivery of their anesthetics.

REFERENCES

1. Finder RL. The art and science of office-based anesthesia in dentistry: a 150-year history. Int Anesthesiol Clin 2003;41(3):1–12.

2. Robert R. Sedation and general anesthesia in oral and maxillofacial surgery: a US perspective. Chapter 6b. In: Andersson L, Kahnberg K-E, Pogrel MA, editors. Oral and maxillofacial surgery. Chichester (West Sussex): Wiley-Blackwell; 2010. p. xxxviii, 1274.

3. Doze VA, Westphal LM, White PF. Comparison of propofol with methohexital for outpatient anesthesia. Anesth Analg 1986;65(11):1189–95.

4. McKeage K, Perry CM. Propofol: a review of its use in intensive care sedation of adults. CNS Drugs 2003;17(4):235–72.

5. Beers R, Camporesi E. Remifentanil update: clinical science and utility. CNS Drugs 2004;18(15):1085–104.

6. Mackenzie N, Grant IS. Comparison of propofol with methohexitone in the provision of anaesthesia for surgery under regional blockade. Br J Anaesth 1985;57(12):1167–72.

7. Rama-Maceiras P, Ferreira TA, Molíns N, et al. Less postoperative nausea and vomiting after propofol + remifentanil versus propofol + fentanyl anaesthesia during plastic surgery. Acta Anaesthesiol Scand 2005;49(3):305–11.

8. Mortero RF, Clark LD, Tolan MM, et al. The effects of small-dose ketamine on propofol sedation: respiration, postoperative mood, perception, cognition, and pain. Anesth Analg 2001;92(6):1465–9.

9. Jacobs JR, Glass PS, Reves JG. Technology for continuous infusion in anesthesia. Int Anesthesiol Clin 1991;29(4):39–52.

10. Olivier P, D'Attellis N, Sirieix D, et al. Continuous infusion versus bolus administration of sufentanil and midazolam for mitral valve surgery. J Cardiothorac Vasc Anesth 1999;13(1):3–8.

11. White PF. Clinical uses of intravenous anesthetic and analgesic infusions. Anesth Analg 1989;68(2):161–71.

12. Bailey JM. Context-sensitive half-times: what are they and how valuable are they in anaesthesiology? Clin Pharmacokinet 2002;41(11):793–9.

13. Miller DR. Intravenous infusion anaesthesia and delivery devices. Can J Anaesth 1994;41(7):639–51 [quiz: 651–2].

14. Robert RC, Liu S, Patel C, et al. Advancements in office-based anesthesia in oral and maxillofacial surgery. Atlas Oral Maxillofac Surg Clin North Am 2013;21(2):139–65.

15. Hillier S, Mazurek M. Monitored anaesthesia care. Chapter 31. In: Barash PG, Stoelting RK, Cahalan MK, et al, editors. Clinical anesthesia. Sixth edition. Philadelphia: Lippincott Williams and Wilkins; 2009. p. 815–32, 1760.

16. Hogue CW, Bowdle TA, O'leary C, et al. A multicenter evaluation of total intravenous anesthesia with remifentanil and propofol for elective inpatient surgery. Anesth Analg 1996;83(2):279–85.

17. Jacobs JR, Reves JG, Glass PS. Rationale and technique for continuous infusions in anesthesia. Int Anesthesiol Clin 1991;29(4):23–38.

18. Candelaria LM, Smith RK. Propofol infusion technique for outpatient general anesthesia. J Oral Maxillofac Surg 1995;53(2):124–8 [discussion: 129–30].

19. Bennett J, Shafer DM, Efaw D, et al. Incremental bolus versus a continuous infusion of propofol for deep sedation/general anesthesia during dentoalveolar surgery. J Oral Maxillofac Surg 1998;56(9):1049–53 [discussion: 1053–4].

20. Wright PJ, Dundee JW. Attitudes to intravenous infusion anaesthesia. Anaesthesia 1982;37(12):1209–13.

21. Cooper L, Nossaman B. Medication errors in anesthesia: a review. Int Anesthesiol Clin 2013;51(1):1–12.

22. Jensen LS, Merry AF, Webster CS, et al. Evidence-based strategies for preventing drug administration errors during anaesthesia. Anaesthesia 2004;59(5):493–504.

23. Lonnqvist PA. How continuous are continuous drug infusions? Intensive Care Med 2000;26(6):660–1.

24. White PF, Eng M. Fast-track anesthetic techniques for ambulatory surgery. Curr Opin Anaesthesiol 2007;20(6):545–57.

25. Taylor E, Ghouri AF, White PF. Midazolam in combination with propofol for sedation during local anesthesia. J Clin Anesth 1992;4(3):213–6.

26. Kodaka M, Suzuki T, Maeyama A, et al. Gender differences between predicted and measured propofol C(P50) for loss of consciousness. J Clin Anesth 2006;18(7):486–9.

Printed and bound by CPI Group (UK) Ltd, Croydon, CR0 4YY

08/05/2025

01864711-0005